STAR SIGN SLIMMING

JUNE BAKER-HOWARD

STAR SIGN SLIMMING

metro

Published by Metro Publishing Ltd, 3 Bramber Court,
2 Bramber Road, London W14 9PB, England

British Library Cataloguing in Publication Data. A CIP
record of this book is available on request from the British
Library.

ISBN 1 84358 057 8

1 3 5 7 9 10 8 6 4 2

Design by ENVY

Printed and bound in Great Britain by Bookmarque

Papers used by Metro Publishing Ltd are natural,
recyclable products made from wood grown in sustainable forests.
The manufacturing processes conform to the environmental
regulations of the country of origin.

Contents

Foreword

I have written *Star Sign Slimming* so that you can use astrological principals to your advantage. Astrology offers the opportunity to gain self-knowledge and therefore a greater self-understanding.

One of the basic rules of Astrology is 'everything is true to its moment of time', so your horoscope or astrological birth chart shows the energy pattern present at the time you entered the world and, therefore, tells much about the structure of your own energy mass and, what I like to call, your 'inner dynamics'.

An awareness of these inner dynamics, including your inner strengths and potential weaknesses, is as vital to the success of any slimming campaign as it is to achieving goals in business or work-related situations, or in your important personal life. Once you become familiar with the predispositions of your zodiac sign, you will be able to apply this knowledge in ways that help you stay more in control of your actions and responses, and, therefore, of your weight and shape.

It is said that our bodies are the chariots for our souls, so it is the responsibility of each of us to try to keep out particular chariot in good shape, without carrying so much excess weight around that we are slowed down. Follow the guidelines given in this book and you should be able to succeed in your slimming efforts, even if other diets have failed.

THE SUN SIGNS – Do you know yours?

There are twelve signs recognised in modern astrology. (Once there were more than twelve!) **Your Sun sign, also known as your star sign, birth sign or zodiac sign is** the most important factor in the judgement of your birth chart because it represents conscious behaviour and your life's potential. It is the real you! The very essence of you, and it is determined by the moment you took your first independent breath.

By tradition and observation, certain personality traits are attributed to each of the signs. The positive traits should be regarded as the potential of the individual and the characteristics that must be developed in order to find true fulfilment. The negative traits can hold you back in life and some of them could become obstacles of the kind that make it hard for you to lose weight.

The sign under which you were born never changes, so it is your sign all through your life. However, the Sun doesn't enter or leave each of the signs of the zodiac at the same time or even on the same day each year, which is why the dates used in the star columns that I write for newspapers and magazines are only approximate.

In my experience some people are completely

wrong about their Sun sign and were born under a different sign to the one they have claimed as their own. The moment of truth has come as a shock to certain of my readers.

If you were born on the cusp, i.e. around the time of the month when the Sun left one sign to enter another, you would normally have to consult an ephemeris, which is a timetable of the planets, in order to establish your true Sun sign. However, a time table has been provided in the last section of this book. This covers the years from 1920 until 1990. If you are unsure of your birth sign, simply refer to these. You could be in for a surprise and find that you were born under a different Sun sign to the one imagined.

Here's wishing you every success with your slimming campaign.

JUNE BAKER-HOWARD

Getting Started

Start by weighing yourself and measuring your vital statistics and make a note of these. You should repeat this exercise each time you complete a seven-day weight loss plan. You should soon feel excited, as well as encouraged, by the results!

Next read the section of this book that applies to your particular birth sign. If you were born on the cusp (i.e. around the time the Sun makes its monthly change of signs, which is known as its ingress) you may need to verify your correct birth sign by referring to the tables provided in the last section of this book.

Your Sun sign belongs to one of four groups, each of which is associated with one of the four elements – these being Fire, Earth, Air and Water. A weight loss plan has been especially created for each group. (For example, Aquarius is an Air sign, and Aquarians will find that the diet suggested for their group will suit their temperament perfectly).

The diets in this book are nutritionally approved and are based on low calorie intake, as well as healthy eating. This means that you can follow an eating pattern that is right for you, and which also results in a loss of weight without a loss of vitality.

THE 12 SIGNS OF THE ZODIAC

ARIES

The Sun's entry into Aries, around the 20th March, heralds the coming of the Spring time in the Northern hemisphere. Aries, which is the first sign of the zodiac, as well as the cardinal (or principal) Fire sign, is symbolised by The Ram – the assertive leader of the flock. Ruled by Mars, the red planet, which was labelled the 'planet of war' by the ancient astrologers, the tendency of Aries people is to initiate action, take control and blaze a fiery trail as they go through life. Mars is also associated with force, passion and energy. Thus the Aries personality possesses a strong desire to lead rather than to follow and, above all, to see results. Aries is a sign of both courage and enterprise.

YOUR SLIMMING PERSONALITY

The Key word for your sign, one which sums up your go-ahead personality beautifully, is action. An ideal slimming philosophy!

You are a positive thinker and, like the Ram, the symbol of Aries, you tend to tackle life's problems head on. This means that you will soon get to grips with your weight problems.

What is more, as a Fire sign, you are quickly

SINFUL SUGAR
Adding sugar to drinks and cereals is strictly forbidden, and a habit your waistline can do without, so start now to retrain your taste buds. Challenge yourself to stick to the first week of your diets completely sugar-less. It becomes easier as you go along and you'll end up loathing the sickly sweetness you used to love.

motivated and ready to act, but must learn to sustain a steady and constant flame when it comes to dieting, rather than burning yourself out in a sudden bright but short-lived blaze of enthusiastic slimming.

Your leadership qualities equip you to inspire others because you capture their imagination with your confident manner and your energy. It is the fiery element within you that urges you to make your mark on the world, and make others aware of your presence.

Even in childhood and throughout your teenage years your tendency to make decisions for yourself, combined with the sheer strength of your will, must have made you a power to be reckoned with. Your ability to take control can at times be completely misunderstood however, and seen as a sign of rebelliousness or a refusal to accept authority. Muster the force of your will-power now and you will soon lose your surplus weight because there's little that can stand in your way when you have committed yourself to a definite plan of action. Your aim in life should be to make good use of the force of your will, which is, indeed, one of the most wonderful assets you could have when it comes to slimming.

YOUR SLIMMING STRENGTHS

The ambitious, assertive side of you, which likes to win, is one of your main slimming strengths. Another is that you firmly believe that we all make our own luck in life and regard effort as a vital ingredient in any cake of success. You truly expect to succeed in whatever you start. It's also likely that you possess a determined and brave side to your personality and rely on your own experiences rather than those of other people, so you'll almost certainly keep an open mind about slimming the astrological way until you've tried it out for yourself.

Where dieting is concerned, you possess a considerable advantage over many of the less decisive signs of the zodiac and those who are unable to carry through their ideas. Your spirit, your drive and your willingness to try out something new – all these mean that you are able to grasp the essentials of a dieting routine and make it work for you. As a decision-maker, you have already confirmed your intention to slim. You did so when you purchased this book! What is more, your speed at forming judgements means that you're unlikely to waste a single day, now that you have decided to go ahead.

You are ready to work hard to feel proud of the way that you look, so can be fairly ruthless with yourself if needs be, this is particularly the case when you realise that your body isn't as slim and supple as it used to be or should be. In common with other people born under your dynamic sign, you are self-motivated and self-disciplined, with the will-power to battle on until you are totally satisfied with your overall appearance. You do like to be in control at all

times, but especially of your figure and appetite, and
no matter how painful, you are not one to fool yourself
about your vital statistics, or what needs to be lost in
the way of weight or dimensions. This is because it is
in your very nature to face up to problems.

BONUS POINTS

You achieve most when you have a goal to work towards.
It's possible your parents cashed in on this fact when you
were young, by offering you sweets or ice cream for being
good. Use this strategy yourself by promises yourself a
new hairdo or outfit when you achieve your target weight,
or even a holiday to show off your new and supple shape.

If you're true to your Sun sign, it is important for
you to make an impact and show others that you
possess a clearly defined sense of identity. Have you
noticed how you like to wear black or strong,
attention-claiming colours? This is your way of
saying "notice me". It follows that you rarely do go
unnoticed – another good reason to ensure that your
image never lets you down.

Fortunately, it's rarely necessary for you to need a
prop, so it will not worry you unduly if you have to
follow the diets in this book on your own, even if
means eating different meals to those of your family
or companions. In fact, you often prefer to play a lone
hand in life so that you can do things in your own
decisive way. The truth is you can resent it if someone
tries to influence what you put on your plate, or
attempts to impose their likes or dislikes onto you.
You certainly possess the strength of character to give
up any food item that turns out to be damaging to
your health or figure.

One of your gifts is the convincing way you have of selling anything you believe in, or intend to try out for yourself so don't be too astonished if your friends, colleagues or other members of your household indicate that they want to follow your lead and do something positive towards resolving their own weight or figure problems.

YOUR SLIMMING WEAKNESSES

One of the root causes of your figure problems is likely to spring from a hurried life-style. Especially as fast food often consists of fattening and filling snacks, such as chips, hamburgers and doughnuts – the type of temptation that eases hunger pains but piles on the pounds.

It will assist your slimming efforts if you learn to plan your meals in advance, so that you avoid placing yourself in a position where you are suddenly hungry without the appropriate calorie-controlled meal available. Also, never go without food for long periods because you find it difficult to cope with that awful sinking feeling, which goes right down to the pit of your stomach, causing your best intentions to fly out of the window.

You are often the person who initiates new projects, but it is only too easy for you to lose interest if progress is slow, or if there are too many boring details to contend with. Learning to have patience and to wait for results is not only essential to your personal development, it's very necessary if you are to slim successfully, so be warned that crash diets can reduce your weight in the short term, but tend to add it on with a vengeance in the long-term. This is because your body goes into its survival programme whenever its fuel tanks are depleted. Not only do your hunger pains increase, because your body is urging you to increase your intake as quickly as possible, (to refill your fatty cells which are being used up), but your metabolism slows down at the same time, so you actually start to function on less calories than you did originally.

IN THE RAW
You hate to be kept waiting when you're hungry but there's no need to wait for ages to prepare a meal, or to cook first before you eat. Dishing up salads and vegetables in the raw, just as nature intended, is especially good for you and none of the nutrients are cooked out. Peeling skins off loses vital vitamins – particularly Vitamin C.

Ironically the very qualities that can so often bring you success, can also incline you to take risks or the sort of short cuts, that more cautious or less adventurous souls would resist. The desire to see quick results in whatever you start is one of your greatest slimming obstacles because it will be easy for you to become discouraged or impatient, if your bathroom scales, or tape measure, fail to come up with the right answers within the expected time-scale.

There is also a rebellious side to your nature, that doesn't take kindly to too many rules, which could conflict with the fact that to stay slim requires a regular and sensible eating pattern, one which not only provides you with sufficient vitamins and nutrients to deal with the stresses and strains of everyday life, but which also leaves you with enough energy to enjoy an active leisure time. Insufficient nourishment caused by trying to speed up your weight loss can make you tense, irritable and even difficult to live with. The weight loss plan given for the fire signs is ideal for your go ahead personality.

In your battle against overweight – and this is a battle well worth fighting, both for the sake of your health and also for the pleasure you derive in knowing that you look good – you must curb your Aries impatience and take your diet one day at a time.

Ignoring the warning signs can also be one of the contributing factors for an Aries weight problem. Sadly, many an Aries has only decided to slim, or taken an active interest in their health, when the damage has already become obvious.

YOU AND YOUR BODY

You are more body conscious than most. A natural pride in your appearance and keeping fit, means that you are prepared to invest time, money and effort into achieving the weight and the shape that makes you feel good about yourself. It's hardly surprising that Aries is considered to be one of the most energetic signs of the zodiac because your inclination is to take instant action as and when a problem arises. Although this inner drive will get you off to a flying start when

---

DO-IT-YOURSELF

As you tend to be a 'do-it-yourselfer', try adding your own touch as a banana, fresh strawberries or any selection of chopped or pureed fruits to plain yoghurt, (the low-fat variety of course) to make a mouth-watering dessert. You'll enjoy it all the more knowing that you used your imagination and prepared it yourself.

TEMPTATION ON WHEELS
You like to be mobile but resist the temptation to fill up your car with a selection of mints, chocolates, sweets or other 'goodies' in order to combat the boredom of long sessions sitting behind the wheel. It's only too easy for hours spent driving or stuck in frustrating traffic jams to result in a spare tyre – one of the fatty sort – right round your middle.

it comes to dieting, it is vital to pace yourself. It would be counter-productive to expect too much, too soon.

When faced with opposition your instinctive desire is to attack in one way or another. This means that you have to cope with anger and the resultant adrenalin pouring into your blood stream, which can sometimes put you off your food, only to bring your appetite back with a vengeance when life has quietened down again. You can also fall into the trap of eating or drinking too much through turning any anger or upset you feel on to yourself, thereby venting your frustration on your body.

Exercise is an essential part of any slimming plan for you and you need to find adequate physical outlets for your pent-up energy. Regular exercise keeps you feeling fit and ready to take on the world. Work-outs, weight lifting and activities which allow you to channel any anger, annoyance, aggression or frustration in a healthy way, are ideal. An exercise machine is likely to be one of the best gifts that anyone ever buys you!

Aries people have the reputation for being headstrong, so it's hardly surprising that the head, brain and eyes are the parts of the body particularly associated with your sign. The symbol of Aries represents the horns of the Ram, another indication that the traits of Aries are recognised as being forceful and insistent, sometimes to the point of being pushy or acting like a battering-ram.

Coming to terms with yourself and with the life you have created is part of your recipe for perfect health because your body soon reacts to the way you feel inwardly. When you're unwell, you can usually identify the underlying reason. This is often connected with a loss of control in some way because you are a person who puts great store in being in control of your life. It is when you feel that your hands are tied and you cannot take the action you would like, or you find yourself in a situation where others are making all the rules or issuing all the orders, that you are most likely to overeat or become ill, or depressed.

YOU AND YOUR EMOTIONS

Whether you realise it or not, you are usually the one to set the pace in your emotional relationships. Even when you were a small child, it's likely that you made the rules in the playground with your brothers and sisters. Your unwillingness to compromise in life means you will rarely share your time with people who annoy you or bore you. You insist on total loyalty from your friends, family and partner and there have to be powerful reason before you will give a second chance to those who hurt you, reject you or let you down in any way.

You make an enthusiastic lover or friend, and once you give your heart you are more than prepared to fulfil the fiery promise of your sign. What you seek above all is proof! Proof that you are loved and needed. You have to be certain of your partner's affections. Because of this deep rooted need, you hesitate to put yourself in a position where you could become hurt or snubbed. This means that you sometimes don't put as much effort as you could with regards to cultivating new friendships.

Although you tend to be happy with your own company, you are even happier when you know that there's a partner waiting in the background, – someone who is ready to show you appreciation, which brings out the best in you. You can feel very lonely if you're deprived of company for long periods.

Your reactions are instantaneous, so you're best avoiding moody or unreasonable people. Anger is one emotion that can make you break your diet in a flash. Don't vent your rage by demolishing the contents of a plate of sizzling fish and chips, or a steaming dish of curry. Wait until you have calmed down and assessed the situation. Otherwise it could be too late to consider the damaging implications your upset has had for your figure.

Other people cannot fail to be aware of you and they are attracted to you by your air of confidence. However, only diet together with another person if they are prepared to play a supportive role or are keen to follow your lead.

Your feelings are stronger than you sometimes care to admit or show, as you like to put on a brave front. It is not always easy for you to live up to the dynamic reputation of your Sun sign. Only too often you must find that other people look to you to do their dirty work and make their excuses and complaints, mistaking your brave facade for nerves of steel, not realising that you too can be anxious or unsure of yourself. Once you have achieved your desired weight you are certain to be told by those who don't know you well, that "of course it was easy for you".

You relate particularly well to other Fire signs, Aries like yourself, or Leos or Sagittarius. Not only do you benefit from the mutual understanding that exists between all of the Fire people but you are motivated and stimulated by the competitive element that is sparked off between you, even when you are the best of friends. This competitiveness can provide a tremendous boost in a shared slimming campaign and could be the challenge that is needed if ever your will-power is in danger of weakening.

If there are Water-sign people in your life – Cancers, Scorpios or Pisces, beware of their effect on your diet! They are so sensitive that they will "feel for you" and react to your hunger the instant they hear your stomach rumbling. A Water sign will probably urge you to eat – albeit in the name of loving and caring. All Water signs tend to express their affection and friendship by looking after other people, which usually includes offering lashings of food, regardless of whether or not it's really wanted. Unfortunately, rejection of their hospitality can often be taken as a rejection of themselves. You can avoid hurting your Water-partner or friend's feelings however, if you appeal to their natural compassion and under-standing. Explain gently just how important it is to you to become slim and healthy and they will soon be helping, instead of hindering you.

Those born under Gemini, Libra and Aquarius,

these are the Air signs, will appreciate the reasons behind your desire to lose weight and they will probably supply you with a long list of additional reasons for dieting. Even so, they'll prefer to let YOU start dieting first to see what happens. Once you have reported back to them with the pros and cons, they are likely to follow suit. Air and Fire people are very compatible, so usually achieve excellent results when they join forces in a project. The cool, detached objectivity of an Air person helps you to see pitfalls that you could miss in your haste, while in return you give them enthusiasm and encouragement.

The three Earth signs, Taurus, Virgo and Capricorn could prove to be either your greatest allies or your greatest source of frustration. Their down-to-earth, common sense attitudes will help you to plan and structure your life, so that your imaginative ideas stand more chance of bearing fruit. Conversely, their caution and insistence of taking one step at a time, could cause you to miss your moment.

Earth people are keenly aware of the importance of food, which they tend to view as a source of pleasure, as well as survival. Try to benefit from an Earth person's ability to organise ahead because you could find dieting that much easier generally if an Earth-partner or friend supervises your meals. However, unless you persuade them to share your diet programme, you'll find your determination is constantly tested by the sight and smell of the tasty food that Earth people seem to love preparing.

YOUR CREATIVE ENERGIES

You attack your hobbies with as much enthusiasm as

> **DAWDLING DANGERS**
> Avoid dining out with a Libra, unless you're not especially hungry, because it could be your undoing diet-wise. While they are dithering over the menu, you will have scooped up the nuts, crisps, olives or bread rolls, and any other tempting titbits designed to stimulate your appetite.

any other area of your life, so often excel in whatever you put your mind to accomplish. Aries tend to walk off with many of the prizes when they enter competitions. However, you're unlikely to compete unless you feel that there's a strong chance of winning because you hate to be second best. Slimming is one competition in which you're guaranteed a prize – That is providing you stick to the rules and follow your diet. In common with the other two Fire signs, Leo and Sagittarius, it's a matter of pride to you to be good at anything you undertake.

In off-duty moments, you like to be busy. You can be tremendously productive, providing that you steer clear of projects that drag on for too long or which cannot hold your interest. Instead, concentrate your energies on activities that excite and enthuse you, so that you don't eat out of boredom. It is to your advantage to plan your spare time in such a way that you are never at a loose end.

You're usually attracted to leisure interests that have a useful side and often develop a range of skills as you go through life. Mars, your planetary ruler, is associated with iron and many Aries are adept at working with metal. Engineering and mechanics are typical Aries occupations and even the most feminine Aries tends to be a deft hand with screw-driver and spanner.

Work is one of your prime outlets for creative expression and you put you heart and soul into whatever you do, acting as your own severest judge and critic. The frustration you feel when a job goes wrong, can lead you to finding solace in a snack outside of eating hours. This is a good reason for you to be realistic when assessing the length of time required to complete whatever you've started.

When you feel the urge to take a holiday, your first instinct is to start packing – this can even be before you have actually booked your trip or decided on your destination! Your ideal location has to hold a few surprises and a degree of the unknown, as well as plenty to do and see. The chances are you would find it hard to be stranded in a very quiet location for very long. A new venue every year would suit your style and love of adventure. If you are a typical Aries, you enjoy a challenge, as well as lots of bustle and activity. After all, your keyword is ACTION – the reason why you have what it takes to make a successful slimmer.

TAURUS

20th APRIL TO 20th MAY

TAURUS, the second sign of the zodiac, is symbolised by the Bull and thus associated with strength and fertility, as well as the staying power attributed to the Taurus personality.

Taurus is ruled by the lovely planet Venus, the planet of love and harmony. Weather permitting, Venus is often visible in the sky around the time of sunset, so is called the Evening Star. Taurus is the "fixed" (or steadfast) Earth sign and the need for stability, and security, is a driving force in all Taureans.

YOUR SLIMMING PERSONALITY

It is natural for you to like good food and wine, because yours is a sign associated with a love of gracious living. Many Taureans are blessed with hearty appetites, having the ability to eat anything from pickled onions, baked beans, toasted cheese sandwiches, profiteroles and after dinner mints, all at the same meal – without feeling uncomfortable or suffering from the slightest hint of indigestion. Fortunately, slimming doesn't mean that you'll be deprived of all eating pleasures because the diets planned for you in this book allow you to enjoy one or two luxuries and yet lose weight at the same time.

You are very well aware of the attractive person you can be when your measurements are in proportion to your height because you have a good eye for line and also for colour. This, plus your love of beauty makes you an ideal candidate for slimming because it is particularly distressing to you if your appearance doesn't match up to your own high standards.

Taureans are reputed to be the gardeners of the zodiac and when you plant seeds, they usually flourish because you are gifted with the diligence and the patience to allow them to grow in their own good time. You also enjoy the rewards of your labour in other areas of your life and, where slimming is concerned, you can use your qualities of perseverance and strength to bring the reward of a new, slimmer and healthier you.

YOUR SLIMMING STRENGTHS

Once you have decided to pursue a certain course of action, you rarely abandon it because you have the great gift of persistence, which enables you to work slowly but surely towards your goal. This willingness to

---

GROW MORE

As Taureans are considered the farmers of the zodiac, it's highly probable that you possess 'green fingers', the hallmark of a good gardener, so why not grow your own salads, tomatoes and other natural produce? The satisfaction of eating home-grown, low calorie and health giving fresh food, that you planted and cared for yourself, even in a window box, will make slimming all the more enjoyable.

apply yourself and stay with your plans is one of your winning attributes when it comes to losing weight.

You are good at organising both yourself and also others, especially children. When you establish a routine, you ensure it can be followed without too much inconvenience or hassle, so your family tends to go along with your well regulated pattern of living.

Being practical, determined and sometimes even stubborn is one of your greatest slimming strengths, because you are unlikely to break your diet easily, even if you have a large amount of weight to lose. You are sensible enough to accept that there is no magic formula for slimming and that the only certain way there is of losing weight and staying slim, is to eat less and take regular exercise.

You tend to prefer set meal times, which can be used to your advantage in your efforts to shed inches because it enables you to keep a better control on your food intake than those who follow erratic eating patterns. Taureans, both men and women, are usually excellent homemakers and housekeepers, and it comes naturally to you to do the shopping and plan the meals. However, you are now preparing to begin a new way of life, which is a slim and healthy way of life, so this is the perfect time to review and rewrite your weekly shopping list for food.

It will soon become automatic for you to measure the portions carefully before putting your food on your plate in order to monitor your daily food consumption. It is by retraining yourself to follow new, healthy, slim ways of eating that you'll achieve the shape you'd like to be and, as importantly, retain it.

Most Taureans have a well-developed sense of

humour, one of the finest qualities anyone can possess. This ability you have to laugh at yourself, as well as at life generally, is a definite bonus for you as a would-be slimmer. It helps you to see how ridiculous it is to allow the dictates of your stomach to become over-important.

You usually know exactly what it is that you want out of life and can be charming and persuasive, or blunt, demanding and outspoken, as the occasion demands. A good indication that you have what it takes to talk others round to your way of thinking, which will help you gain support for your slimming campaign

YOUR SLIMMING WEAKNESSES

Ideally, you should have been born rich, because you have gourmet tastes. If you can't afford the caviar and champagne lifestyle that you would like, you may be tempted to compensate by awarding yourself generous portions of rich foods. This may excite your taste buds but unfortunately it also serves to whet your appetite, so that you want even more. As you well know food provides you with essential fuel for your body, but any surplus eaten is processed and stored by your

SLOWLY DOES IT

Satisfaction can take time to register, so get into the habit of eating slowly. If you're very hungry, eat a small starter to take the edge off your appetite, then wait ten minutes before attacking the main course. If you serve your food up on a smaller plate than the size you are accustomed to, you'll leave the table feeling as if you've had a full size meal.

body as fat. However unwelcome this fact may be, you can only lose weight by either reducing your calorific intake, or finding a way to increase your output of energy, which almost certainly means a change in your dietary and exercise habits. Even so, a love of good food is as natural to you as breathing and many Taureans are tip-top cooks and wonderful hosts and hostesses. This appreciation of the culinary arts and entertaining must be controlled carefully as it is often one of the contributing factors to you putting on weight.

GOURMET CONTROL

You've a taste for the very best in food and wine. There is nothing wrong with this providing you are aware of which 'bests' are the most fattening and ration these to very special and important occasions. In fact, 'moderation in all things' should be your motto because your body will use what it needs and then convert any surplus fuel into fat.

Your waistline and hips tend to suffer if you indulge in too much socialising, so parties, weekends away and holidays pose a formidable threat to your figure.

At the same time, others tend to turn to you in times of trouble because you possess a certain aura of peace and calm, even when the opposite applies. Your hospitable nature and kind heart can encourage you to console your loved ones with reassuring plates of comforting food, but as you like to put others at their ease, you often join them in eating it, at the expense of your figure!

If you are confronted with a sudden change in your routine, you are inclined to resist it because you dislike upheaval and do not welcome too much excitement or disruption. You can also be extremely suspicious of anything that's untried and untested. This can make you miss out when progress depends on adapting to new methods. Your reluctance to experiment can tie you to traditional but solid eating habits that gradually make you gain weight, without you always being aware of it. That is, until you have a problem! The diet for Earth signs in this book has been carefully adapted with your personality in mind. You will find it easy to comply with them, once you have accepted the changes that must be made.

YOU AND YOUR BODY

Taureans stand more chance of reaching a ripe old age than any other sign of the zodiac. Statistics prove that there are an unexpectedly high proportion of those born under the sign of the Bull amongst the over-eighties. Indeed, if you're a typical Taurean, you're blessed with a strong and robust constitution. However, you will probably have to work hard at keeping it in shape, especially as you grow older, because your liking for good food and a comfortable

GETTING ABOUT

As Taurus is considered a 'fixed' or steadfast sign, it's especially essential for you to get up and get moving. Although this diet will work if you stay with it, you will help things along and improve your overall shape by taking some exercise every day. Walk, play sport, swim, dig the garden or buy a tape and limber up. But if you join a keep-fit class, beware of the out of class socials!

lifestyle are often totally at odds with your body's true requirements.

As the parts of the body associated with Taurus are the neck, throat and chin, your neck is one of your high risk areas for storing fat. You should always keep a careful watch on your chin-line and take immediate dieting action if you notice any developing signs of a double-chin.

You will find that the gentler forms of exercise suit you best. This is preferably taken at regular times and intervals. Yoga and walking are ideal as they allow you to tone up your body gently and keep it supple, without too much effort or discomfort.

Moderation is a key factor in achieving the slimmer lines you seek, so plan to exercise every day rather than saving up your good intentions for a grand slam once a week. It's important for you to enjoy exercising and also to know with certainty that the end result will be worth the time and energy you expend.

Ruled by the planet Venus, associated with the Goddess of love, most Taureans, especially the female members of this sign, are very attractive to the opposite sex. No doubt you grew from being a bonny, bouncing baby, to a good-looking teenager without giving your good fortune a second thought. Sadly, it is often only after you have allowed your weight to creep up and your figure to lose its ideal shape, that you recognise the necessity for regular weight-watching. Dieting and taking regular exercise are the only way you will be certain of retaining the shapely figure that is rightfully yours. The diets given in this book will make it easy for you to do just this. They also take into account your Taurean appreciation of

QUICK FREEZE

Why not prepare your own ready-frozen, calorie counted meals? It will not only save money and time, it will help you change your eating habits and attitudes to what constitutes a sensible meal. You could batch cook some of your most successful diet-meals – those that work for you because you particularly like them. Then label them and freeze them for future use.

good food and enjoyment of creative cooking, as well as your liking for entertaining.

It cannot be emphasised too strongly how essential it is for you constantly to keep your eye on your weight and to adjust your daily diet accordingly. This should be a way of life for you if you want to stay slim. Beside the obvious health risks associated with being overweight, feeling ungainly makes you miserable and lethargic.

YOU AND YOUR EMOTIONS

You're a romantic, chasing ideals and sometimes placing others on a pedestal. To your friends and the ones you love, you are a tower of strength. When you enter into an emotional commitment, you do so with a passion and the conviction that it will last, and no power on earth will put you off the one you have chosen. Ideally you need an insurance policy against getting hurt emotionally because, if ever your faith is proved unfounded or misplaced, it can be extremely bad news for your figure!

It is rare for you to rush into a new liaison because you prefer to get to know people gradually before allowing them to grow too close. You need to feel comfortable and relaxed with your partner at all times. As you are a person of commitment, you also need someone who reassures you and makes you feel secure, someone you can respect and admire. Your Taurean passion can quickly turn to scorn if the object of your affection fails to live up to your expectations. Any disturbance of your emotions can produce disturbed eating patterns.

Personal relationships are a serious matter to you because it is essential for you to have harmony in your home and in your leisure time. You are often the hub of the household and usually have ready access to the food store, which can be a slimming obstacle. You are a fairly resolute character, but remember that your way is not necessarily the only way. Allow the other members of your family or household to have their say in the way things are run. You may learn a new trick or two by paying attention to what they say and watching what they do. Particularly take note of the slimmer members of your household, who are probably naturally following the advice given in this book.

As a friend you are the "salt of the earth" type that is staunch, loyal and totally reliable; but you can come unstuck by expecting too much from those you care about, so the ability to accept other people as they are is important for your emotional tranquillity. Loving someone goes hand in hand with having pleasure in your book because you shower the person you care about with thoughtful gifts and compliments, as well as good food.

Other people love to pin the labels of being "stubborn and possessive" upon Taureans, but you're not as unmovable as some might think. (You can now

prove this by successfully completing your diet plan.)
Your natural caution means you will be standing
strong after those who jump too hastily have come
unstuck. Don't allow your, often commendable,
reluctance to stop you now, because as a child of the
planet Venus, beauty and attraction are your gift by
birth-right, a wonderful reason for making the
decision to diet.

You feel at ease with those born under the other Earth
signs, Virgo and Capricorn, as well as other Taureans.
However, tread carefully when it comes to eating
together, because a common tendency for all Earth
people is to equate food with comfort. Even so, Earth
people can help to keep you on the right track if they
have pledged their support to you. Your attitudes to life
and also to eating, are very similar to theirs, so they
will understand and sympathise with your problems.

There is usually a natural empathy between you and
the people born under the Water signs of Cancer,
Scorpio and Pisces, who are very sensitive to your
needs and to your feelings. Water people can be much
stronger and tougher than they appear, so don't
hesitate to team up with a Water friend or partner in
your slimming campaign. They will help you to keep
going! As Water signs are also very sensitive to their
own bodies, they can teach you how to tune into your
own and make you more aware of the signals your
body is constantly sending to you.

Most Water people possess a natural gift to heal
and soothe others in times of trouble. You can
confidently turn to your Water friends when you are
feeling tense and so avoid taking your frustrations
out on a plate of food.

The intensity and the sheer energy you put into your emotional relationships can be overwhelming for Air people, who value detachment, space and the freedom to come and go as they please. The Air sign individuals you come into contact with, whether they be your close relatives, your partner or your colleagues at work, are certain to approach the whole question of slimming from a different angle to yourself. The reason why they eat can be as much for something to do, as to meet their basic survival needs and energy requirements. Don't expect them to be especially sympathetic to your diet efforts because they are as different to you as chalk is from cheese. The rules and time tables that work so well for you will probably be an anathema to them.

Life should never be dull with a person born under a Fire sign, whether that Fire sign be Aries, Leo or Sagittarius, because their warmth, enthusiasm and ability to enjoy life will stimulate you and encourage you to be adventurous. However, as all Fire sign people tend to hold strong views of their own, don't be surprised if there is an occasional

---

DANGER ZONES

Never go shopping for food when you're even the slightest bit hungry because the delicious aroma of freshly baked bread or roasted coffee beans can make your stomach turn somersaults and your will power cave in. Delicatessens and up-market super-markets are highly dangerous zones when you are ready for a meal. Only enter them if you've eaten already and are well armed with a carefully thought-out list. Even better, send someone else to buy the weekly groceries!

clash of wills between you. Nevertheless, they are just what is needed to give you a push if ever you're stuck in a weight-rut. They can also motivate you to do something about it instantly if ever your bathroom scales begin to creep up past your desired weight limit.

YOUR CREATIVE ENERGIES

Anticipation is a large part of the pleasure you derive from all leisure activities. Like all Earth people, you're good at organising and planning. When you start a project, you expect to see it through to the end, and you take great pride in your accomplishments. Whether you involve yourself in a business venture or a spare time interest, you spend a long time thinking it through before you start and your eye for detail usually ensures that the end result is perfect or as perfect as it can be! You are one of the most colour-conscious signs of the zodiac and painting, whether with canvas and easel or a paint tin and step ladder is a wonderful way for you to channel your creative energies. Most Taureans excel at art and interior design and Taureans are well represented in the world of fashion and beauty.

MANY FAMOUS SINGERS ARE BORN UNDER YOUR SIGN, so it's likely that you adore music and singing and you may even possess a good or powerful singing voice yourself. Music stirs your emotions and nourishes your soul. Fortunately, it is harmless to your figure! In fact, it can do you a power of good health-wise if you combine music with dance or exercise, at a class or along with a video tape.

There's a peaceful, quiet side to you, which thoroughly enjoys curling up with a good book. Apart from reading purely for pleasure, you're also an avid reader of D.I.Y. books as they satisfy the productive side of your personality. Your personal library may well include subjects such as 'how to paint in oils', 'how to landscape your garden' or grow bonsai trees, and it's a fair bet that cook books occupy a great deal of shelf space in your home. For many Taureans food is a favourite hobby.

Pleasant, unhurried and stress-free holidays represent a passport to delight for you. Time spent in the countryside has special value and meaning to you because being close to nature revitalises you and helps you to feel at peace with the outer world, as well as within. You hate hardship, however, so may opt to go without a summer vacation, rather than settle for leaving the comforts of your own home to stay in accommodation that's not really up to scratch.

There is scarcely a Taurean who doesn't grow plants, bulbs, flowers, cacti, radishes, prize marrows, and other interesting species of vegetation. There's an endless list! You possess a natural empathy with the earth and can usually tap into the life source of the vegetable kingdom, often producing quite magical or beautiful results.

Above all, there is one thing that can stand you in good stead in your campaign to lose weight. It is your appreciation of beauty, because it lifts your spirits when you like what you see when you look at yourself in the mirror. Think of your weight loss plan as a steady road to a beautifully proportioned you, which will assist the flowering of your inner personality.

GEMINI

21st MAY TO 20th JUNE

GEMINI, the third sign of the zodiac, governs the period of the transition of spring time to summer in the northern hemisphere.

In the heavens, the constellation of Gemini contains two very bright stars, Pollux and Castor. Hence the idea that Gemini is a dual sign. This duality is also indicated by the glyph of the sign, the Roman numeral II–representing the two sides of the Gemini personality, male and female, extrovert and introvert, and quiet and talkative. Mercury, which is the closest planet to the Sun and also the fastest moving planet in our zodiac, is the ruler of Gemini, and a mutable (or moving) Air sign. The urge to move freely from place to place is a driving force in those born under this sign, as is the need to communicate.

YOUR SLIMMING PERSONALITY

There is a friendly, outgoing and active you, and also a quiet and more thoughtful you. You are not brazen, but you are not shy either. In fact there are two completely different sides to your personality. To slim successfully you must learn to cater for both, because the opposing elements within you sometimes urge you to try to "have your cake and eat it", which you may manage to get away with at times, but not when it comes to dieting, as your figure will soon remind you.

Life usually forces you to make many choices. This may between two people, two jobs or two interests, because your life plan, as a Gemini, is designed so that you can learn to choose wisely. When you do, you find success. This will soon be apparent when you try to slim, because your choice of food will soon influence whether you are slim and dynamic, or sluggish and overweight. In this instance your choice should be an easy one to make because no true Gemini ever likes to look old for their years.

Like the wind, blowing through the trees, you need to be free to change direction at whim, and it is likely that you are quick in both thought and action and find yourself constantly on the move. No doubt you have always been anxious to live life to the full and be youthful forever. You hope to extend the summer-time of your days as long as possible, often refusing to accept the idea that you will ever look old. Your zest for life and your desire to enjoy as many different experiences as possible, has earned your sign the label 'the butterfly of the zodiac'. Your liking for variety and your ability to quickly flit from one activity to another will help you to follow this weight loss plan successfully.

Quick-silver, a liquid metal which possesses the property of responding instantly to changes in temperature, is also called Mercury, so it is to be expected that your temperament as a Gemini and one of Mercury's children, should also reflect this ability to react in a flash to external stimuli. You are the kind of person who tends to take on more than one thing at a time, changing your activity to suit your mood. Follow the diets given in this book with confidence because they have been created with this liking for flexibility in mind.

YOUR SLIMMING STRENGTHS

A heartening thought for you is that Gemini is essentially a "slim" sign and also a youthful one. Many Geminis look and act much younger than their years, with a lightness of step and a brightness of eye that makes the Gemini man, or woman, whatever their age, an attractive and vital person. The problem of overweight is in fact an uncommon one for Geminis because your restless energy provides you with the means to stay slim and retain a youthful figure. This knowledge should encourage you to stick to your diet, because once you have succeeded in your slimming campaign and reached your target weight, your zodiac temperament, combined with your new self-awareness, should see to it that you remain slim, with only the occasional need to check your eating habits.

Geminis are ruled by their minds rather than their emotions, so it follows that once you have talked yourself into taking positive action to resolve your overweight problem, you are already half-way towards achieving success. In fact, your mind needs to be

---

SLIMMING-TALK

Talking, which tends to be your main mode of self-expression, is a wonderful aid to losing weight. Therefore if you suddenly feel all alone, seek the company of a friend or relative or catch up on your telephone calls rather than fining consolation in food. Your disposition particularly likes a sounding board – someone who gives you a feedback on how they think you're doing.

supplied with a constant supply of food for thought. Fortunately, this is better for your slimming campaign than supplying a constant supply of food to your body, via your palate!

You rationalise and analyse carefully every scrap of information that is presented to you, so will appreciate the medical reasons as well as the cosmetic ones for retaining a healthy weight.

The fact that a wide range of interests attracts you can be used to your advantage because you have the ability to find enough worthwhile distractions to take your mind off food. A never ending interest in anything that's new or novel, or that happens to be the current vogue or out-of-the-ordinary, means that you will be ahead of others in trying out your weight loss plan. At the same time you'll enjoy talking about it to your friends.

If you're typical of your Sun sign, your mind is an active one, with a natural curiosity in anything and everything. Even as a child you probably exhausted your parents and teachers with questions beginning with "Why", "How", "What" and "When". This "child-like" inquisitiveness is likely to continue throughout your life and represents a natural strength where

---

MASTERMINDING

You will find it easier to avoid over-eating if you become immersed in the sort of projects that stretch your mind, so swat up on politics, computer skills, antiques, weather patterns and health matters or even the state of the economy. This will help to keep the pointer on your bathroom scales from zooming up.

slimming is concerned. Your healthy interest in what's happening in the world at large, and in what motivates other people and makes them tick, helps you to stay young. It also allows you to switch your mind off the sort of problems that drive those who are more pedestrian in their way of thinking to seek their answers in food and drink.

Your great gift of versatility can be utilised in another way to assist in reducing your weight. You can combine dieting and exercise and still fit in the thousand and one jobs and activities that you usually have on the go, without any of them suffering. Your love of being active makes staying fit especially desirable, because aches, pains and bodily twinges are rarely your favourite topic of conversation.

When you commit yourself to a project, you expect it to work, and to work quickly. You live for the moment, rather than the past or the future, so you require results NOW! TODAY! and IMMEDIATELY! You will appreciate the fact that you can throw yourself into your slimming campaign knowing with certainty that you will soon be enjoying the slimmer you. As you begin your diet you will have taken a very definite and important step towards regaining that slim and fit look that is the true reflection of the inner you. This is a wonderful incentive for you to sort out and plan your food cupboards ready to start your diet with a flourish.

YOUR SLIMMING WEAKNESSES
You collect people with as much enthusiasm as schoolboys put into collecting postage stamps or football programmes. This means that over the years,

GO TO WORK ON AN EGG

Have you ever tried a cold omelette? It makes a surprisingly substantial meal. On days when eggs are included in your diet, why not make one with your low-fat spread allowance and serve it cold. You can vary this theme by adding a selection of vegetables as a filling. Serve with a salad – or even between two slices of bread as a sandwich.

your circle of friends is inclined to increase rather than diminish. You are at your best when you are in one of your frequent sociable moods, surrounded by an appreciative audience. You rarely pass by an opportunity to socialise, especially if it provides the chance to go somewhere new. Here lies your greatest slimming weakness, as eating out can be detrimental to your figure.

Another slimming hazard, so far as you're concerned, is your healthy interest in all that's new or different because if a new type of food or drink comes out on the market, you are probably one of the first to try it. It is essential to be aware of the negative side of your readiness to experiment. Unusual recipes, such as foreign cuisine, can prove irresistible to you and you are usually game to try anything, such as a spicy pizza or well-filled vol-au-vent, at least once. The risk to your figure is twice as high if what you're sampling has the makings of being an entertaining talking point.

As already mentioned, Gemini is a mutable or moving Air sign, so it is usual for you to be on the move. As a busy, active person, it's essential for you to become familiar with the foods allowed in your diet, as well as the quantities permissible because, when you find yourself under pressure or dashing about from one place to another, it's only too easy for you to grab an instant snack, one that's readily available. In fact, it is the small nibbles that represent your Achilles heel. Eating too many quick snacks, which are often high in calories or deficient in nutrition, is a serious slimming obstacle

It's highly probable that you sometimes start to nibble purely because for the reason that you lack something to do which holds your interest. Finding enough mental stimulus is all-important for you if you are to avoid eating out of restlessness and frustration, so plan to change your surroundings and vary your routine whenever you detect early warning signs of boredom. When your mind starts to wander to thoughts of food in between meals, change the subject. Turn on the television, read a good book, start decorating your lounge or go somewhere where there's no food to hand. Even better, begin an exercise session because this will keep both your mind and body busy working towards a profitable goal, i.e, your desired weight and shape. Mini-snacks are permitted only if they are part of your permitted daily weight loss plan as given in this book.

PICTURE PROOF

When you've slimmed right down to your target size, ask a friend to take a photograph of you – then keep it with you wherever you go. Look at it every time you sit down to eat, just to remind yourself what you stand to lose if you over-indulge. All the foods in your weight loss plan are calorie-kind to you and nutritious into the bargain.

YOU AND YOUR BODY

It is your abundant enthusiasm for both work and play that keeps you young at heart, so it follows that your appearance should reflect the exuberant inner you, this is the you that is slim, attractive and eternally youthful. It is not easy for you to accept that you're overweight, as it rarely feels natural to you for your body to be too fat or out of shape.

Your innermost urge is to communicate, so your body language is usually fairly expressive, which is all the more reason to ensure that you are not giving out the wrong messages due to you being overweight or out of breath.

Regular exercise is essential to you and does wonders for your state of mind and confidence, as well as your circulation, muscle tone and overall shape. Stretching your body and limbering up helps you to combat stress and mental fatigue, and also keeps you slim and supple. This is an important point to remember because your lively restlessness can sometimes take its toll on your nervous system. Having adequate rest periods and correctly balanced meals are vital if you are to feel in peak condition, so establishing a good set of eating and exercise habits is all important.

The hands, the arms and the nervous system are the parts of the body particularly associated with Gemini. No doubt you gesticulate or "talk" with your hands, which are rarely still. You find it stressful if you are forced to stay immobile for long periods and in fact rarely sit still for long in your everyday life. When you take exercise, it should be of the fun variety, easy to do and sociable in nature, and preferably of the type that

SWEET EXCHANGES

Look out for breakfast cereals based on oats, which provide a healthy alternative to muesli and bran as listed in your weight loss plan. It's important to avoid sugar-coated or sweetened cereals, but if you really miss sugar on them, try a substitute or a sprinkling of dried fruit instead. Also substitute yogurt for milk, so that you can save your milk allowance for drinks later in the day.

can be done out of doors in the fresh air. Cycling, dancing, gardening and keep fit classes are all likely to appeal to your healthy desire to stay active. Team up with like-minded friends to take exercise and you'll find it twice as rewarding because you will also be able to satisfy your liking for congenial company.

Even so, do allow adequate time for the more serious, introvert side of your nature, because periods of peace and quiet are essential for you. These must be balanced with those of a more lively nature to ensure that you stay in good spirits and in harmony with yourself. Your conflicting needs should never be ignored because being aware of your own complex personality is an important part of your personal healthy living programme. On the one hand, too much exposure to hustle and bustle and too many claims on your resources exhaust you, and causes you to lose your sparkle and "joie de vivre", while on the other hand, too much solitude and lack of stimulus depresses you and drags you down.

A splendid tip for healthy living is to give yourself regular breaks between tasks. Ten minutes relaxation before you charge off on a new assignment could do you more good than any tonic that comes out of a bottle.

YOU AND YOUR EMOTIONS

Flirting is traditionally considered to be a favourite pastime for a Gemini. Whether or not this is one of your pleasures, there is no doubt that those born under the sign of Gemini do hold a great deal of sex appeal. All the more reason for you to keep a regular check on your weight. You are exhilarated by the glamour and excitement of an initial attraction but have to guard against boredom creeping in when you are in a long-term relationship.

You seek a lively, versatile and resourceful partner, one who is well informed and on your wavelength. He or she should also be as intelligent as you because you soon become bored with anyone who is dull or has little to say for themselves. You tend to keep the various parts of your life in separate compartments, so can sometimes fail to give your most important personal relationships as much time and attention as they merit.

You are a thinker, who is inclined to live in your head and often find it difficult to keep your mind off any problems that has become urgent or is likely to arise in the near future. Generally, you prefer to stay in control of your moods and feelings at all times, and you like other people to do the same. This means that you usually try to avoid anyone who makes too many emotional demands, especially as you find it hard to cope with heavy, intense scenes or floods of tears.

Even so, you seem to be fatally attracted to the sensitive Water sign people, Cancers, Scorpios and Pisces because they have what you lack, which is a natural awareness of their own feelings and emotions, which you sometimes suppress. You are opposites in every way. You form judgements by using reason and logic: Water signs do so through their impressions and feelings. You are analytical and detached, and they tend to accept life at face value and be subjective. (Nothing can infuriate you more than a Water sign person's ability to come up with the right answers for what you consider to be the wrong reasons!) If you are trying to diet, don't let a Water sign invite you for a meal because they will take your refusal of food as a personal rejection, and you know how you hate a scene! Better to enlist their sympathy and support by explaining the situation beforehand.

In common with your fellow Air sign people (the others are Librans and Aquarians) you need freedom of movement and personal space, and the right to follow your own interests. A relationship with someone born under an Air sign stands a good chance of working out for you because your needs are similar. An Air partner or friend will respect your desire for privacy and will also be in tune with you mentally. Like you, they arrive at conclusions by thinking things through in a logical sequence, and are not unduly swayed by emotional or sentimental arguments. Slimming with an Air partner will prove mutually beneficial to you both because you'll be able to talk each other through the moments of temptation and keep dieting and food matters in perspective.

People born under Aries, Leo and Sagittarius, the three Fire signs, are extremely compatible with Gemini. Fire people inspire you with their flair and their boldness. You can usually spot any flaws in their imaginative ideas and help them to succeed. However, their bluntness can sometimes offend you. This trait

---

FREE RANGE

You need the freedom to do your own thing as much as possible, which means that your weight loss plan will suit your temperament. You can eat your food in any order you wish, and you can swap your meals around to suit your changing appetite or preferences. If you keep a close watch on what you consume in the working day, you will be able to indulge yourself a little in the evenings and when socialising, without threatening your waistline.

---

can be useful for your slimming attempts as you can count on honesty if you ask for their opinion of your problem areas. They have an uncanny knack of getting straight to the root cause of a matter.

Earth people, those born under Taurus, Virgo and Capricorn, deal in realities, while you deal in possibilities and probabilities. They call a spade a spade and fat FAT, while you prefer to examine the reasons WHY you've added inches, and consider the cause as important as the effect. A close relationship with an Earth person can help you put structure into your arguments. At the same time you can encourage them to be more flexible in their way of thinking. You'll impress an Earth partner or friend most by showing them that you, like them, can wait for results. As they believe in facts rather than speculation tell them to keep watching your figure.

YOUR CREATIVE ENERGIES

Anything new, novel or different appeals to you, so when you choose a venue for a special night out, it is likely to be to see the latest film or play or to try out a new eating-place or disco. Bright lights and plenty of action suit the bill, particularly if they provide plenty of material for future discussions. Dinner parties, cabarets, pantomimes, any function that provides interesting personalities and stimulation – these are all for you. Any excuse to meet up with your friends is enough to set you organising drinks, snacks, suppers or tea and biscuits. Your Gemini willingness to sit and chat can pose a problem if you're dieting as you may find that you're nibbling your way through the afternoon or the evening.

Nevertheless, bringing people together is one of your greatest delights, especially if they are unlikely to meet each other in their normal social spheres. It's probable you attract a varied selection of people to your side because there is nothing you enjoy more than listening to different points of view, in fact the more unusual or controversial the conversation the better. Divide the time you spend on leisure activities between those projects you can do on your own and those that involve other people. In this way you will satisfy the two different sides of yourself, which means that you can expect to be twice as pleased once you have achieved your ideal weight. You are probably happiest with a number of hobbies because your desire to learn is one of your greatest motivations. Evening class, discussion groups, workshops, books and the whole range of practical and scientific programmes offered through computers, television, videos and films are tailor-made for Geminis.

You are a communicator who takes in information and passes it on in one form or another: if you join up with others to slim, you will soon be happily swapping tips and encouraging others to follow your good example. Indeed, the company of convivial friends is as vital to your well being as the air that you breathe. Luckily, if you're typical of your Sun sign, you find that striking up new acquaintances and relationships comes easily to you. The outward-going side of you is the one that most impresses others. It is because of this, that yours is considered to be one of the most friendly and gregarious signs of the zodiac. Your very ease with words and your ready wit equips you to teach, sell and handle others confidently.

Your nervous reactions tend to be quick and you may be adept at working with your hands. You are usually better at mental pursuits than dealing with heavy physical tasks. You stand more chance of being happy and, therefore healthy and slim, if your occupation and your lifestyle allows you freedom of movement.

CANCER

June 21st to July 22nd

Although the sign of Cancer is the cardinal (or principal) Water sign, it happens to be the least conspicuous sign of the zodiac.

Cancer, the fourth sign of the zodiac, is symbolised by The Crab, although in Egyptian times it was called the Scarab. Like a crab there is a soft, vulnerable side of the Cancerian nature, which is often hidden under a thick defensive shell. Ruled by the Moon, which controls the tides and all fluids on Earth, there does seem to be an ebb and flow to the Cancerian personality, who tends to feel bright and full of energy on the Full Moon, but quieter and more withdrawn when the Moon is waning. Cancer is the sign of the Mother and homemaker, in so much as it embodies the need to nurture and look after others.

YOUR SLIMMING PERSONALITY

Your first slimming task is to learn to say 'No' when others offer you food. Not because you're a greedy person – Cancer is not a particularly self-indulgent sign – but because you are reluctant to hurt someone else's feelings. Ask yourself this question. As a child did you try hard to eat up all your food you were given, even if you weren't hungry, just to please your mother or those who cared for you? The answer is almost certain to be 'Yes' because as a Cancerian you're extremely sensitive to others. Even now, when you're eating with your friends, family or partner, you may find it difficult to wave away the dessert or second helping of a delicious meal that has been cooked especially for you.

You often have strong feelings of guilt when you need to refuse a gesture of love or friendship. This Cancerian trait of saying 'Yes' in order to please others makes it easy for you to put on unwanted pounds and inches when you're sharing food and drink with those you like or care about. The more sociable and friendly the mood, the greater the risk is to your figure.

YOUR SLIMMING STRENGTHS

You can use your Cancerian sensitivity to work out the best way to refuse unwanted food without causing offence to others. A white lie, such as, ' I have already eaten or I had a big breakfast or lunch and couldn't manage another mouthful' may be easier than explaining that you are trying to lose weight. This

---

WEIGHING IN

Cancerians often love to cook but must remember that portion control CAN'T be done by guess-work.

Do buy a set of scales on which you can measure precise ounces or pounds or their metric equivalent. Continue to use them until you can recognise the right amount of food without error. Buy a set of measuring spoons too – these will help you to avoid unwanted calories as you cook.

BE PREPARED

Preparing meals for the family can be a tempting exercise for you, so try to organise your time so that you can deal with this task when you've just eaten. That way, you won't want to nibble whatever it is you are making. Wrap and refrigerate, or freeze prepared food until it's wanted and you'll be less tempted to pick at it.

especially applies if you are in the company of tubby but well-meaning friends who regard your diet plan as unnecessary. When you are with those who want what's best for you, enlist their help and support. You'll experience the feelings of love and security that are so important to you when you know others are on your side, helping you achieve your goal.

Nevertheless, you may have to eat alone for at least one meal each day if you are to stick to your weight loss plan because, as you probably know only too well, the cooking of attractive and satisfying meals for your family, or the one who matters most in your life, is one of your favourite (and sometimes most fattening) way of expressing your love. Although you rarely enjoy eating alone, turn this to your advantage because it will prevent you from lingering over the meal table, and serving yourself another helping of dinner or dessert.

One great advantage you have is your wonderful Cancerian quality of tenacity. You rarely give up once you have set your sights on a target. Your tremendous persistence can carry you through when other would-be slimmers are giving up. Use this gift throughout your slimming campaign and you will achieve your desired weight and shape. Even if you hit a time when you consider you are faltering in your diet, call upon that tenacity to keep on trying. You are sure to win through in the end. Make no mistake, you are more than capable of achieving the goal you have set yourself. Your sign is famous for its ability to "stay with it" no matter what it takes.

Another advantage of your sign is your special sensitivity to the twenty-nine day lunar cycles; so make a note of the dates of the New and Full Moons that occur each month. They are particularly important to you when trying to lose weight, or following any kind of keep-fit regime.

The day of the Full Moon and the day before it, are the best days of any month for you to begin any new diet, or to start again if necessary. Your chances of offloading surplus pounds quickly are then at a peak. (You should also choose the time around the Full Moon to free yourself from any other unwanted habits, such as smoking.) It's likely that you will restless and unsettled around the time of the new Moon, so will benefit from taking up a new interest, especially if it enables you to channel any pent-up energy into a worthwhile goal.

YOUR SLIMMING WEAKNESSES

It's not for nothing that Cancer is considered the sign of the World Mother. One of the main ways in which you can find fulfilment in life revolves around looking after other people, belonging to a unit and 'mothering' the people you care about.

That word 'Mother', so frequently associated with your sign, sums up your strong urge to nourish, nurture and care for the other people in your life. Your

SOCIAL SLIMMING

You are a wonderful hostess but your dinners, or parties, can sometimes lead to your own undoing! It's best not to entertain when you're on a diet, unless you can adapt a diet meal to suit the tastes of your guests. Try to keep your own portions controlled and never put temptation in your own way by preparing high-calorie foods.

first instinct, when someone enters your home, is likely to be to feed them, whether you do so by offering them a cup of tea or coffee and a biscuit or a full-scale meal. This represents one of the obstacles in the way of you achieving your target weight and keeping it. The satisfaction you feel from sharing food, you've so lovingly prepared for your family or guests, can quickly undo all the good work of a week's careful dieting. Your figure is equally at risk when you accept hospitality, especially when the person who presses you to 'just have another drink' or 'just finish this last slice' is a loving friend or relative. Your key to success lies in understanding this side of your nature.

Any concern shown for your well-being is usually warmly received on your part. This is because you delight and truly appreciate being pampered and fussed over, and being made to feel special. Deep down in the recesses of your subconscious mind, you equate caring with security and are reminded of either the safety, warmth, love and attachment of your early years, or of the loving care you somehow missed out on and have therefore searched for all of your life.

Indeed you can cope with an unlimited supply of love, so if love and affection are being offered to you

---

NIFTY NIBBLING

If you do want to eat between meals, be clever by dipping into your next meal in advance rather than eating extra bits and pieces. A slice of fruit, or a mouthful of fresh raw salad vegetables will appease any hunger pains and keep you on the straight and narrow, diet-wise.

---

in the form of food and nourishment, it isn't easy for you to refuse. This means you sometimes accept meals or drinks when you're not really hungry. Apart from any other consideration, your natural sensitivity and understanding of others means that it is not your way to offend your prospective host or hostess by rejecting the gesture of goodwill and friendship that has been kindly offered.

YOU AND YOUR BODY

As a Cancerian you are especially sensitive to the messages your body sends to your brain, even if you sometimes choose to ignore what your body is trying to tell you.

To prove the point, open the door of your refrigerator or food cupboard and imagine eating one of the items on display to see how your body responds. Think about all the possible snacks you could have and ask your body which it most prefers. You could be surprised at the answer. A craving for a particular food can indicate the necessity to top up on essential vitamins or minerals.

What is more, you are usually acutely conscious of the effect that over-eating, drinking, smoking or neglecting to exercise regularly has on your health and your shape. The parts of the body associated with

Cancerians are the midriff, waist and breasts. These are the most vulnerable areas for storing surplus fat.

You should favour the kind of exercise that is enjoyable rather than hard work. If you can rope in a friend to exercise with you, so much the better. Cancer people usually enjoy activities that take them into or close to water. They also like to dance or combine movement with music.

The saying 'prevention is better than cure' is particularly true in your case, because the sight of your own naked body in the mirror, if it is bulging in all the wrong places, can upset you for the day. You tend to be your own severest critic when it comes to your appearance. Keeping a constant eye on your weight and vital statistics is your best strategy to stay slim because the prospect of having to pare off large amounts of excess weight is especially hard for a sensitive Cancer person to bear. Make up your mind always to take immediate action if and when the pointer on your bathroom scales creeps round to your personal danger level

Your personality type is an important factor in your predisposition to certain types of illness, and a key factor in your attitude to food. It is by understanding yourself that you will begin to see why you're the weight and shape you are at the moment. Sometimes a change has to occur within ourselves before we can get to grips with the changes we would like in our outward appearance.

It cannot be emphasised enough that knowing yourself is an important part of being able to maintain a healthy body and positive outlook on life. Learning to acquire an inner state of calm is vital for you to

stay healthy, happy and slim. Constant stress or
anxiety will take its toll on your nervous system and
digestion, and will, eventually, also leave its mark on
the way you look. It is essential to include clearly
defined periods of rest in your programme, even if
that means turning a blind eye to the mountain of
jobs that you seem to attract.

YOU AND YOUR EMOTIONS

Cancer is the leading, or Cardinal, Water sign. The
element of water is associated with sensitivity, feeling
and emotions. This is why your feelings and emotions
always run deep, and this is true whether those
feelings are usually calm and peaceful, or turbulent
and overwhelming. Unfortunately, this means that
your eating patterns can soon be disrupted if you are
upset or worried. You long to be liked, as well as loved
and it is in your nature to put others first, which can
cause you to neglect your own needs and interest. You
can alternate between losing your appetite completely,
due to feeling all 'choked up', to miserably eating your
way through a bout of depression, regardless of the
consequence in terms of unwanted inches or weight.

TENDER TRAPS

Your friends and loved ones pose the greatest threat to
your diet intentions. In particular beware of Leo's love of
pampering others and keep a firm eye on your waistline if
dining with a Taurean, who is likely to be a super cook.
Be extra careful to have eaten, or have the meal prepared,
if you intend to feed an impatient Aries, because the risk
is you will share the appetizers they will want immediately
they arrive in your home.

For these reasons it is important for you to learn to control your eating patterns so that they are consistent, even when your emotions are in a turmoil.

Have you noticed that you sometimes have an inclination to take things too personally? This over sensitivity can cause you unnecessary pain and can even be the underlying reason for any health problems you experience. Your best way to cope, when facing criticism, is to learn to stand back a little and become an observer of life, rather than becoming too involved in every issue.

The ability to detach yourself – to stand back – will go a long way towards helping you to overcome the urge to eat or drink when you are in need of comfort. Also, and this is because of your great need for affection (Cancer is an especially romantic sign) you also need to know how to adjust your slimming efforts so that they do not become a problem in your close relationships.

This will be easiest if your closest friends, family and loved ones were born under Water signs like you were. The people born under the other two Water signs, which are Scorpio and Pisces – share your sensitivity, and you may find that their weight fluctuates just as yours does. It will be ideal, of course, if you can persuade a fellow Water sign to follow the diet along with you. You can rely on a fellow Water sign to understand your moods, and to share your triumphs and elation. Don't be shy, either, about turning to a Water sign for sympathy on days when you the going seems tough.

You should also be able to gain a great deal of comfort from a partner who was born under an Earth sign - Taurus, Virgo or Capricorn. In this case you stand to benefit, not from their sensitivity but from their 'down to earth' approach. Don't be offended if you find that your Earth sign partner or friend tries to cheer you up by offering food or drink (the last thing you need) as comfort. Just explain 'I know you mean well but I shall feel unhappy if I fail to stick to my weight loss plan.' Those born under Earth signs appreciate ambition and determination – even stubbornness – and will like and respect you all the more.

Those both under one of the three Air signs, Gemini, Libra and Aquarius, like to debate and discuss, and may at times undermine your confidence in your weight loss plan by suggesting other, alternative ways to slim – or even tell you it's all in the mind and that you do not need to slim at all. Your best way to deal with them, without upsetting yourself, is to stay calm and appeal to their reason. Say something like: 'I respect your point of view, but this is something I want to try for myself.' If there are Air sign personalities in your life, such as friends, partners or close relatives – you will know that there is also a strong mutual attraction and there is also likely to be a great deal of stimulating conversation or even arguments! Those born under Air signs admire independence, but hate emotional outbursts. If you show them this book you may be helping them to be more like you, able to tune into their own innermost feelings.

Perhaps the most challenging of relationships for a Cancerian is that which exists with any of the three Fire signs: Aries, Leo and Sagittarius. You can

> **MOVE IT!**
> Look on being active as an important part of keeping your weight under control, because you are far more likely to stick to your weight loss plan if you've plenty to do. Resist any tendency to brood on life, when you should be getting out and enjoying it more. Get up, get out and get moving. You'll feel better for it.

sometimes find their energetic and assertive approach to life overwhelming. Nevertheless, it is this very energy and self-confidence that can provide the sort of support you need, so don't hesitate to enlist the help of a Fire sign person when dieting. A Fire sign friend or partner, who also needs to lose weight, would be ideal – and they may add a competitive note to making progress. Follow your individual diets together, and your relationship could blossom, because the qualities of the Fire sign include one or two of those you lack yourself and vice versa!

YOUR CREATIVE ENERGIES

Your slimming programme will be helped by finding time for diversions and activities that keep you pleasurably occupied – and stop you thinking about food. With this in mind, you should plan to indulge in the hobbies, and even the holidays, that are right for Cancer people.

Although the popular myth of a Cancer native is one of domesticity, you demand far more from life than washing dishes and doing domestic repairs. It is essential for you to have an absorbing interest, independent of other people. Unlike many other signs or the Zodiac, you are quite capable of keeping more than one project on the go at a time, knowing they all stand a real chance of being completed.

Cancer is a very creative sign, so you may be good at many different forms of creative expression, cooking, decorating, gardening, interior design, dressmaking, hairdressing, wine making. There's an almost endless list of home crafts you can turn your hand to. You can also do well in other creative pursuits and many Cancerians are inspired writers, poets, musicians and artists. This is because your deep feelings pour into your work and add a meaningful content to it.

Your inspiration tends to be at a high when you are happy and full of the joys of life. When you feel a creative mood coming on, you should try to take advantage of it! It gives you intense satisfaction to produce a tangible result from your imagination, and any thoughts about nibbling food or of sipping drinks disappear like magic when you are keen to finish a project you've started.

Your ability to immerse yourself completely in whatever it is you are doing, is one of your greatest assets when it comes to losing weight. In fact, your antidote to over-eating could be to throw yourself whole-heartedly into a new interest. Do this and the hours will slip by unnoticed before someone else's demands for food, or sheer hunger, reminds you that it's time to eat.

You can usually keep yourself occupied and may take your leisure activities extremely seriously. Many Cancerians earn money from their hobbies, either by establishing a profitable sideline, or by turning a favourite hobby into a career or business.

You enjoy being organised by someone else, providing they do it efficiently. Indeed, you warmly appreciate those who exhibit good organising skills, especially if they combine them with plenty of imagination. However, Cancer is one of the four Cardinal Signs – which means you are a leader at heart and happiest when you are active. Your perfect holiday must include something to do, other than just lazing around, especially as holidays tend to be one of the more hazardous times for your figure. The truth is moments of boredom encourage you to over-eat. Being near or on, the water soothes and heals you, whether you are strolling along a river bank or sailing on the sea.

LEO

23rd JULY TO 22nd AUGUST

The sign of Leo, which is symbolised by the Lion, the powerful king of the jungle, governs one of the hottest astrological months in the northern hemisphere.

Leo, the fifth sign of the zodiac, is ruled by the Sun, the centre of our solar system as well as the prime source of light and heat. Associated with the element of Fire the constellation of Leo is very noticeable in the night sky. Bright and therefore easy to spot, it acts as a strong indication that those born under this sign tend to stand out in a crowd. The Leo personality is motivated by a burning desire to prove itself and to initiate action.

YOUR SLIMMING PERSONALITY

The state of your figure often reflects your current ambitions. You throw yourself whole-heartedly into any cause which fires your imagination and that is the time when you're less inclined to depend on edible props to get you through each day. As a Leo it is especially easy for you to be noticed and remembered. However, although you know how to steal the limelight, at times you also need to disappear quietly into the background and this is when you may be tempted to have a snack too many. A pity, because when you do make an appearance, it is important for your self-esteem to know that you look good and that your figure is able to stand up to close scrutiny.

The Sun is the ruler of your sign, and like the sun you have an inner need to shine and be appreciated. Your need of approval is a vital point to remember, so look forward to basking in the respect you will earn from your friends and family by proving that you have the will-power to slim down to the supple, lithe being that is really you. This well-earned respect will encourage you to make your new way of eating and drinking, your norm.

As the "fixed" fire sign, you are bound to use this slimming book with enthusiasm. Once you believe in anything, you rarely waiver or change your mind. The "fixed" quality of Leo equips you with a sense of loyalty to a cause or a belief. You would not be reading this book if you had not already made up your mind that it holds exciting possibilities. Indeed, when you open this book there is no doubt you will be tucked away somewhere on your own, wishing to investigate it before you admit to anyone else that you have read it. It is usually all or nothing with you, and if you like what you read, not only will you recommend this book to others, it will also be high on your list as a special gift for your friends and family members.

YOUR SLIMMING STRENGTHS

Pride in yourself and the way you look represents one of your greatest strengths so far as staying slim and healthy is concerned. The knowledge that you can

MEDICAL TIP

If you have any kind of physical heart problem, it goes
without saying that you should consult your doctor before
changing your diet. However, if you're suffering from a
heart ache of the emotional sort, it may pay you to
consult your best friend rather than trying to 'doctor'
yourself with a comforting éclair or a large gin and tonic!

dress up in smart, trendy clothes that make an
impact, whenever you like without feeling
embarrassed about your shape, is the perfect
incentive for you to lose weight when necessary. It is
well worth working for the reward of being able to
show off your new, slim profile. Criticism is also a
wonderful spur to you to improve your image.
Although someone else's chance remark can dent
your ego, it can act like a trigger to set you off on a
determined fitness or slimming course.

Even as a child, your parents and teachers must
have had to handle you with respect because your
strong will and ability to stick to your guns means
that you only budge when it suits you to do so. You
cannot fail to succeed in your efforts to slim if you
muster this will-power now and keep your ultimate
goal clearly in sight. Your resolute nature and
determination, as well as the diets in this book,
provide the winning formula to slim, so set yourself a
realistic target weight today.

Another one of your qualities, which is your self-
discipline, is a great slimming strength and just what's
required for you to stick to a steady and effective
routine. Never doubt that you can achieve the weight
loss you seek, because the stubborn side of your

COVER-UPS

When buying new clothes, be firm with yourself and resist buying loose garments that camouflage your flab. Instead shop for the style you would really like to wear, even if you are bulging at the seams for the first few weeks of your diet. That Leo pride will act like a spur to your efforts to lose weight and soon have you streamlined all over.

---

personality will help you here. Even in one short week you will be able to see and feel the benefits.

When you put your mind to it, you excel in the art of persuasion so should have no difficulty in coaxing your family and friends to support your efforts to look after your body, which is one of your greatest assets.

You tend to dress up or dress down, with no half measures, more often than not according to the shape of your figure. Therefore it is important to stay in control of your weight when you regain your desired size. Once you begin your diet programme, you will have taken a very positive step towards doing something for yourself. By all means enlist the support and encouragement of your friends and other members of your household, but don't worry if you have to go it alone, because you have reserves of courage, which you may not recognise. The company of other people is good for Leo morale, but bear in mind that it is up to you to set the pace.

Leos, both men and women, are good organisers and leaders of others so turn this organising flair to your advantage by planning a healthy diet for the whole family, "adjusting" the size of the portions accordingly. You have high ideals and the power to inspire others to work for you and with you. But all your leadership and drive can be wasted unless you establish a direction and have a clear-cut plan. Make your plan one that is beneficial to your health and one that will also boost your confidence.

You possess a certain dignity and usually appear very self-assured, which makes you a natural manager, teacher and director of operations. You must now review your life-style, even if it results in a total restructure of your shopping and eating habits. The part of you that quite likes to impress will be delighted when you can display your slimming achievements!

YOUR SLIMMING WEAKNESSES

Born in late July or August, you are ruled by the Sun, so rarely feel at your best when the weather is cold or depressing. The winter-time represents one of the most dangerous periods for your figure. Resist the tendency to turn to hot soup and stodgy but filling food for warmth and comfort, if the temperature has dropped to below zero. Exercise is a far healthier way to warm up. Wrapping up against chilly winds and icy blasts will also stop your stomach demanding food, which is nature's way of making sure you put on a protective coating of insulating but unsightly fat.

HIDDEN FATTENERS
As a Leo, you like to eat in style, so be extra cautious about those apparently inoffensive nibbles that many restaurants serve while you're waiting. Salty snacks in particular cause you to want to eat and drink even more. Ask how meat or fish has been cooked and opt for grilled rather than fried every time. Rich sauces or gravies and oily dressings are also bad news.

Unfortunately, this is likely to still be with you when the climate becomes more amicable.

You tend to be a creature of habit; which is fine if your habits are healthy ones and you have consciously and wisely selected them, but beware if they're not! Your habitual eating habits can be the direct cause of a progressive weight gain. Think back to when you were young and ask yourself whether you have allowed yourself to become accustomed to a style of eating which suited your heftier ancestors, but is gradually filling you out so that you are beginning to resemble the fatter members of your family. Keep a note of every single morsel you consume and you would probably be surprised at how often you eat or drink without being genuinely hungry or thirsty.

There is a generosity of spirit that is particular to Leos. This expansive, big-hearted characteristic can be another slimming obstacle because when you entertain, you do so grandly and in style. Only the best is good enough for your family and friends and you go for quality as well as quantity. You must be particularly careful when celebrating or enjoying a special meal because the happy mood of the moment

---

WHAT'S YOURS?

If you like a drink, be crafty and learn a few clever slimming dodges. Make yours a Spritzer, which is a mixture of white wine and soda water-highly, which has far less calories than a straight glass of wine. Low calorie mixers should be the rule if you drink spirits. Also favour low calorie lemonade or cola and opt for a small glass rather than a large one. Bottled mineral water may also appeal, and it isn't fattening!

could prove to be your undoing later if it causes an unwanted weight gain. Treat your body with as much care and consideration as you do your friends. After all, you'll be together for a long time. Pretend you are entertaining one of your most valued friends and they are on a diet. You know how to impress others but you stand to gain most by trying to impress yourself.

The "fixed" quality of Leo provides you with a stubborn streak, which can make you resistant to change, even when it's good for you. Don't dig your heel in now, because there's only one way to attain that figure you've set your heart on and that is by changing your eating habits in fact this could be the best change you've ever made.

Gold, which is Leo's metal, is used in the making of crowns a sign of Leo's ruler ship qualities. No one knows as well as you do that you were born for great things. This can make you want the lion's share of the cake; another obstacle to overcome where slimming is concerned.

YOU AND YOUR BODY

The heart and spine are the parts of the body particularly associated with Leo and problems of the heart, whether physical or emotional, invariably cause your weight to go haywire. Similarly, damage to your back or carrying too heavy an emotional load in the way of problems can also have an adverse effect on your figure. Yet your body is really your pride and joy and the better it looks, the better you feel, so to stay in peak condition is especially important to you.

You respond positively to the sun's warm rays, which revitalise you and put you on top of the world,

SAFE SHOPPING

Many Leos love to shop, so you will have to watch your shopping routine when you feel hungry. At the supermarket, take a basket rather than a trolley if you intend to buy a few items only. In this way you'll resist the temptation to buy on impulse. If you must stop for a refresher in the coffee shop or wine bar, order a mineral water or diet drink.

so gaining a sun tan can provide a great boost to your health as well as your morale. Just be sure to use a sunscreen cream.

You have the capacity to put your whole heart into everything you do and are proud of the way you look, therefore do not resent spending any money and time on keeping yourself in tip-top condition.

There's nothing like being presented with firm evidence of the true state of your figure to motivate you to slim down to the shape you once were, or have always wanted to be. Set diets suit you best and because you can handle a challenge you can aim for and achieve spectacular results in record time.

Weigh in and measure your vital statistics at the same time each week your waist, bust (or chest) and your hips and record them in your own slimming diary.

Your fixed, fiery Leo temperament copes well with a rigid routine when given the right incentive. Leos can become fitness fanatics. This means that when you decide to diet, you stand every chance of achieving your goals in record time. Gymnastics and cat-like exercises, which stretch your body and keep you lithe and supple, are ideal for you. Plan to walk tall and try to be aware of the way you move. Swimming and dancing provide you with the chance to tone up your muscles and relax at the same time, so these are also good for you.

Once you've made up your mind to take positive action, where your body's concerned, there's no stopping you.

YOU AND YOUR EMOTIONS

A loved Leo is a radiant Leo, one who has the ability to spread warmth, joy and sunshine all around. You are able to brighten up the world for others, and this wonderful gift is at a peak when you are in a good emotional relationship. Leo is a Fire sign and you possess a fiery spark within you. This is a spark that can light the way ahead for others. Being without a partner is especially hard for you to bear because you come into your own and do your best work when you have someone by your side.

Your partner's appearance is as important to you as your own, so if they are overweight you will soon tell them to do something about it, which means that you have the perfect excuse to act as a role model.

You prefer to lead rather than follow and like to choose your friends and partners, so usually make the first approach. Although you need time to be on your own, you also like company and to have your fair share of attention and affection. You usually make quite an impression on newcomers. Indeed, a Leo rarely goes unnoticed. It is up to you whether you are remembered for your slim and healthy looks, or for your size.

As much as you hate criticism, asking your opposite number or your best friend for an honest appraisal of your figure could be the motivation to keep you on the straight and narrow with regards to your eating patterns.

Your own ability to be consistent in your affections can lead you to expect the same behaviour from others, and it is hard for you to accept if anyone lets you down. Keeping up a brave front is important to you, so you don't always show it when you feel rebuffed or rejected. This reluctance to pour your heart out and find a shoulder to cry on, even when you have every reason to do so, can be counter-productive for your figure because suppressing hurt feelings poses a threat to your intentions to stick to a diet. You must guard against a tendency to dwell on and magnify problems because when you console yourself with food, you tend to do so in a grand manner, regardless of the consequences for your waistline!

You expect to rule and make no bones about it. Therefore it is worth bearing in mind that although those born under the Water signs Cancers, Scorpios and Pisces, may seem submissive, the opposite is usually the case, so you could experience power struggles, albeit subtle ones, between yourself and Water people. They tend to be masters of manipulation and they, too, want to control and often manage to do so without it being obvious. You are passionate, loyal and a person of commitment, and instinctively respect the depth of feeling that the Water people possess, but be aware that they can dampen your fiery enthusiasm unless you make them feel good about themselves. If you share a diet plan with a Water person and start to lapse, be prepared to be nagged immediately, because little escapes their notice.

You'll have fun with another Fire person in the family. With a Leo, like yourself, or an Aries or Sagittarius, you will spark each other off, so could cause quite a stir. A close relationship with a Fire person should prove to be a lively and eventful one. You share a desire for action with the other Fire signs, so they make wonderful diet companions for you.

You are also well suited in a relationship with someone born under an Air sign. They will both infuriate you with their curiosity and insistence on discussing the whys and wherefores of everything, and fascinate you with a freethinking mind and wealth of ideas. Life with a Gemini, Libra or Aquarius is likely to be interesting and adventurous, and help you broaden your outlook, as well as appraise your eating patterns objectively. Their objective approach to life will stop you exaggerating your slimming problems and help you to see how easy it is to follow your diet and achieve your target weight.

Your ability to be definite, positive and not wishy-washy will go down well with the signs of Taurus, Virgo or Capricorn. These are Earth sign people who

BEST FRIEND TACTICS.

Leos possess the gift of being able to bring the warmth of their Sun sign into the lives of others. However, your urge to entertain with food and drink can be your slimming downfall. If you decide to cheer up a sad Cancerian or a broken-hearted Pisces by making a long friendly 'phone call, make sure that all food items are well out of your reach.

have qualities you admire staying power, as well as practical, common sense. Many Leos team up with them, both on an emotional level and also in business. Announcing your intention to slim and shape up is enough to gain the support of your Earth partner or friends, because it will reinforce their belief in your confidence, which you appear to have even when you are feeling more like a pussy-cat than a lion!

YOUR CREATIVE ENERGIES

Yours is one of the most creative of the twelve signs of the zodiac and it is by developing your potential talents that you become fulfilled and feel true pride in yourself and your accomplishments. Your spare-time activities can provide the creative outlets you need if they are lacking in your work life. You possess a powerful ability to express yourself creatively, and know how to set plans into action and organise events. This power allows you to succeed in many different areas.

You are an individualist and possess a strong sense of drama. Indeed, many actors and entertainers have been born with the Sun in Leo in their birth charts. You need amusements that lighten your spirit. Laughing and making other people laugh represents great slimming boosts because it reinforces your sense of well-being and counters any tendency to make friends with a comforting drink or a plate of nibbles.

You come into your own when you are free to pursue your leisure activities. These should allow you to express your sunny personality. Making music, amateur dramatics, playing games, painting, sketching are all Leo pursuits, but preferably with an appreciative audience to commend your efforts. Involving yourself in activities which are pleasing to you will help you to diet because you will be concentrating on pouring out your energies instead of taking in additional energy in the form of food.

Spur of the moment entertaining is not really your style because you like to plan ahead and usually put careful thought into every detail, from the menu to the way the table is laid. Good presentation is very important to you, so to avoid missing out on the sauces and toppings you like, substitute a low-calorie variety.

Knowing that you can relax completely is an essential part of taking a holiday for you, and even when you go on an activity holiday you tend to allow a couple of days for doing absolutely nothing other than lazing in the sun, preferably on a sandy beach in some exotic part of the world. Invest in some sunshine whenever you can because it lifts your spirits. Aim to make that body of yours a perfect picture, so you'll be proud when you show your holiday snaps to other people.

VIRGO

23rd AUGUST TO 22nd SEPTEMBER

Virgo is symbolised by the Virgin, depicted as a young girl, indicating the untapped resources in Man. And it is by recognising and using their talents to their full potential, that a Virgo becomes fulfilled.

Virgo is one of the three mutable (or adaptable) signs, giving Virgos versatility and also a certain restless quality. However, as Virgo is a one of the stable Earth signs, the Virgo personality also seeks security. Virgo is the sixth sign of the zodiac and the sign of service, so those born under this sign possess an urge to be of value to others, which means they are often found working in supportive roles. The planetary ruler of Virgo is fast moving Mercury, the planet of communication.

YOUR SLIMMING PERSONALITY

Being a Virgo can be exhausting. Similar to a computer, you analyse, sift and store every single scrap of information presented to you. Your ability to observe and not miss the tiniest detail makes you a model slimming candidate and you will be meticulous about following your diet plan.

Virgos are reputed to be the most health-conscious of all the zodiac signs and you have a natural interest in your body and what fuels it. You may be clued up already on calories and food values. Therefore, you will warmly appreciate the winning format of a diet that has taken these into account. Your weight loss programme also caters for your liking for order, which you share with the other Earth signs, Taurus and Capricorn.

You share your ruling planet, Mercury, with the Air sign of Gemini and, like a Gemini, you tend to be restless, and want to be constantly on the move. Unfortunately, no matter how much you move around, you stand as much chance of becoming overweight as any of the other eleven signs! That is why you will benefit from following a structured plan of eating, one that provides you with plenty of energy to meet the demands of your busy, bustling life.

YOUR SLIMMING STRENGTHS

You are a perfectionist with the ability to be your own slave-driver when it comes to correcting any imperfections in the way you look. This is one of your greatest slimming strengths. Losing weight cannot alter your basic body type, the one you have inherited genetically from your ancestors, but by ridding yourself of surplus fat, you can achieve the perfect

---

THINK THIN

As your mind is usually busy considering one thing or another, set yourself a monthly slimming target and be satisfied when you reach it. At times you can expect too much from yourself. Continuously look to future weeks, not days ahead and remind yourself of your ultimate goal whenever you look in the mirror.

HI-TECH SLIMMING

As a Virgo, you appreciate good food, so why not treat yourself to one or two gadgets of the sort that make food preparation as much fun as eating it. Shredders, blenders, graters and slicers will help you enjoy your weight reduction efforts.

---

weight, the one that is right for your height and good for your health.

Another of your strengths is the way you break down large, formidable projects into smaller, more manageable tasks. This helps you to achieve the seemingly impossible, so if you want to change your life, start today, with your weight! And remember that one change invariably leads to another.

The love, the job, the social life you seek, all become one step closer when you know that you radiate confidence. This is the confidence that comes from feeling healthy and looking dynamic.

There is a thrifty side to your nature, which demands value for money. You are sensible enough to know that you must live within your means, so put a lot of thought into how you spend your cash. Fancy trimmings and expensive labels do not fool you because you are a realist, who doesn't judge a book by its cover. You will appreciate the economic sense of only shopping for and eating, what is really needed, rather than buying impulsively in your local delicatessen or supermarket; especially when you see your bank balance grow larger, instead of your waistline.

Virgo, as already mentioned, is one of the most adaptable signs of the zodiac. Your ability to change your ways and your habits to suit the changing demands of your environment, equip you well for following this diet plan. Fortunately, like all Earth signs, you recognise a promising format when you see one. Which is as well because that security-conscious side to your nature needs to know that your chances of success are good. You are also shrewd enough to recognise useful hints, whether they are given intentionally or not, so it will pay you to swap slimming stories with your colleagues, neighbours and friends.

You tend to be a careful person but not over-cautious. You also have staying power, as well as the curiosity to give this new way of dieting the chance it deserves. This will help you to follow each week through conscientiously, until it becomes obvious, as it soon will, that your diet is doing the trick. Although you may dismiss your initial weight loss as a lucky coincidence (because you are not easily impressed) you will be delighted with the fact that once you have slimmed down you can retain your target weight with minimum hassle.

Although, as has already been pointed out, there can be certain drawbacks in your liking for healthy foods, due to the high calorific rate of many products found in a health store, there are also advantages. The interest you have in the workings of your body means that you instantly sense, and are honest with yourself about it, when the food and drink you consume are not doing you any good. Just think how good you'll feel, when you know that every bite you take is exactly what your body needs and a step towards becoming slimmer and more energetic!

> **NIMBLE FINGERS**
> You need spare time activities that occupy your hands as well as your thoughts, or you could soon become very fidgety. The next time you feel tempted to ferret in a bag of nuts or unwrap a packet of ginger-nuts, bear in mind that it's not your stomach but your hands that need to be doing something.

YOUR SLIMMING WEAKNESSES

Those born under your sign are considered to be especially adaptable and flexible, which can be a problem when trying to slim. Your readiness to alter your arrangements at the drop of a hat can result in irregular eating patterns and erratic weight gains and losses, instead of the steady reduction that represents sensible slimming, which is vital if you are to achieve your desired weight loss in the best of health and retain it on the long term.

You are fully aware of the importance of eating sufficient food and not missing too many meals, because you know that no one, not even you, can be effective and function well if they are deprived of nourishment for long periods. However, ask yourself, do you sometimes exist all day on a few cups of black coffee and an apple, only to sit down to a mammoth meal in the evening and then waddle your way to bed? Eating sensible portions of food at regular intervals is essential if you are to slim down your surplus flab and stay slim.

Resolve to avoid stocking up your fuel tanks in one go, especially late in the day. Eating immediately before bed-time is not the way to burn up your fat. A brisk walk after a meal tones up your circulation and

AVOID TEMPTATION

Avoid temptation when shopping for food by making an immediate resolution never to set foot inside a super-market or your local shops again without a list. As a painstaking Virgo, this shouldn't be hard to organise. You should also close your eyes firmly to 'special offers' of the fattening variety. A lower price today could mean a higher weight tomorrow!

allows your body to convert your food to energy more quickly in the process.

Another typical Virgo practice, which is not to be encouraged, is telling yourself that you should eat an extra helping of pie or potatoes in case you have no time to grab a snack later. Not only does this expand your stomach, which then wants more and more, but you also create an unwanted store-cupboard of plump fat cells. However, one of your greatest slimming weaknesses is your reluctance to see good food go to waste, which can prompt you to finish up leftovers, to save them being thrown out if uneaten. You're particularly at risk if raising a young family. Many a young Virgo parent has started a premature middle-aged spread by helping junior out with his, or her, dinner. It may help you if someone else serves the meals and is responsible for removing any tempting tit-bits remaining on the table at the end of a meal.

You like to be well-informed, and have an uncanny knack for assimilating all sorts of facts and figures. No doubt you know more about 'E' numbers, the effects of food colourings and the need your brain has for essential 'B' vitamins, than most of your friends. Nevertheless, even you can fail to appreciate the hidden calories in many of your favourite health foods, especially in pulses, nuts and brown bread. Bear in mind that the size of a portion of food is an unreliable guide to its fattening potential. Your diet will work because it allows you to have bulk without bulges and also eat healthily and enjoy your meals at the same time.

Even if you're not a dedicated party-goer or socialite, you usually have the gift of bringing people together when there's a purpose, so you find yourself the organiser of many events. Your friends and associates are likely to view you as a useful person to know. This means that many invitations to wine, dine and make merry do seem to come your way as you go through life. This can be another obstacle to being able to keep to your weight loss campaign.

In your personal life and your employment, you must try to guard against pressures building up. If for financial, family, or emotional reasons you are unable to organise your affairs in the smooth-running way you prefer, you sometimes take your frustration out on your figure by eating extra to requirements. Remember, your slimming campaign is one area of your life that can follow a predictable pattern and cause no anxiety or aggravations because

LOW COST FLAVOUR

Here's a tip that is sure to appeal to the thrifty side of your Virgo nature. Using a microwave oven takes so little fuel that you can actually save money on your electricity bills. Apart from the economical good sense, you will win by cutting down on those unsavoury smells which waft through your home when cooking fish or vegetables.

your diet has been designed with your personality especially in mind.

YOU AND YOUR BODY

However, your natural interest in body matters is sometimes misunderstood, and may have earned you the undeserved label of being a hypochondriac. In reality, you are usually a fairly healthy sign, with a good chance of living to a ripe old age. Like the other two Earth signs, Taurus and Capricorn, you possess staying-power, which you will need to stick to your diet.

Like Mercury, your ruling planet, it's natural for you to be energetic, which means you are at your healthiest and happiest when you have plenty to keep you occupied. Although yours is a very active sign, you do tend to put on weight, as you grow older, that is unless you are one of those lucky petite, small-boned Virgos, who stay slim all their lives, no matter what they eat. If this is the case, you're more likely to be reading this book out of curiosity than for any other reason!

It is essential for you to learn to relax and accept life as it comes, instead of constantly analysing every potential problem, as well as those that actually exist. Do you find that you leave your home half an hour before you need to, in case you are late? And phone your friends twice in order to double-check your arrangements, sometimes infuriating them in the process? This Virgo trait of checking every minute detail in a plan to make sure that nothing goes wrong, is bound to take its toll on your nervous system.

You can waste a lot of time and effort unless you

learn the power of positive thought. The nerves, abdomen and intestines are the parts of the body particularly associated with Virgo, and yours can act like a barometer to the pressures that build up. Your high standards of perfection can make you worry more than most if your body's size, shape or physical condition is not as it should be. Indeed, possessing a fit, healthy and slim body will raise your morale as well as your vitality.

Following your diet plan will also be a wonderful aid to your digestion. Like your opposite sign in the zodiac, which is Pisces, you may display extremist behaviour when it comes to your eating habits. You can alternate between half-starving yourself one minute, because you are too busy to prepare yourself a meal, and over-indulging yourself the next. Eating the portions suggested in your diet plan will remove any uncertainty you have about how much, or how little, to put on your plate.

In fact moderation in all things is a sound policy for you to adopt. You should aim for a gradual weight loss and take regular exercise. There's no need to be an athlete to exercise your body. In any case aggressive sports and work-outs are not really your style. Generally your exercise plan should lean towards straightforward, repetitive techniques.

Go for the kind of exercise that you can do every day, and may do already in your everyday life, such as walking or cycling. These will assist your weight reduction campaign, and also help to prevent many of the age-related health problems associated with bone and muscle degeneration.

YOU AND YOUR EMOTIONS

Having a partner is important to your sense of security. If you like what you see when you meet someone, you can go to a great deal of trouble to cultivate their company and form a partnership, but you usually think very carefully before making a final commitment. Once you fall in love, you are a person of devotion and will do your utmost to sustain your relationship. You can be misread because on the outside you are cool, calm and unruffled; but on the inside you are warm, earthy and sensual.

Your ability to commit yourself and your sense of dedication can now be applied successfully in your campaign to lose weight.

It is easy for you to make friends because your pleasant manner does not intimidate others. Mercury, the planet of communication, rules your sign, so you are rarely at a loss for words and can strike up a conversation with most people. At the same time you are an attentive listener.

It is in your very nature to try to please others, to back them up, prop them up and protect them from hardship. One of your life's lessons is to learn to discriminate between when help is wanted and when it isn't, because at times your involvement in the problems of others can be counter-productive. To be happy in love, it is important that you feel needed, and have a partner who is not too independent or ungrateful. You are prepared to make sacrifices in order to meet a loved-one's demands. You should now concentrate on pleasing yourself because the right to be in good shape is not only for others. Once you shed your unwanted fat, you could be of service to any overweight member of your circle, by showing them that they, too, can follow the star guide to losing weight.

Casual romance is not really your style because you seek permanency and loyalty from a partner. You are usually extremely tolerant of other people's quirks and failings. Fortunately, as you tend to be a good judge of character, you are rarely taken by surprise. You need someone who will value the many little things you are prepared do to make them happy. It's in your very nature to be obliging and to fetch, carry and fuss over the one who has won your heart. Ideally, they should stimulate you mentally and share your distinctive brand of humour.

Another Virgo, or someone born under Taurus or Capricorn, the other two Earth signs, will appreciate your supportive attitudes and share your liking for a settled existence. This can be a good combination for a life-long relationship and bring few disagreements. However, it could lack the spontaneity and sense of adventure that tends to add a sparkle to life. Trying to lose weight with an Earth partner should go like clockwork because you both accept discipline and rules, especially if you have set your sights on a weight-loss goal.

Teaming up with a Gemini, Libra or Aquarius, these are the three Air signs, brings conflicting aspects into play. They deal in abstracts and theories, while you prefer realities and facts. You can benefit from each other's different approach, whether sharing a home or the fight against flab. You can help them regulate their eating patterns and they can help you forget your worries, and provide you with a thousand and one reasons to press on with your diet.

You will feel comfortable and at home with someone born under one of the three water signs of Cancer, Scorpio or Pisces. They will respond instinctively to you and appreciate your caring qualities. All Water people seek a permanent anchor for their strong emotions so will welcome you with open arms, while you will derive great pleasure from feeling needed or even indispensable. As a slimming team, you will soon find success because the mutual understanding and sympathy that will exist between you will ensure that neither of you buy temptation or place it on the dinner table.

SIPPING STRATEGY
Your diet calls for you to drink 6 - 8 glasses of water a day. (Designer water if you prefer.) Programme this into your daily lifestyle. If you can, sit down as you sip and compile a plan to buy the slim-fit clothes you will need, or the holiday you will take, once you've achieved your slimming goal.

Those born under one of the Fire signs of Aries, Leo or Sagittarius are poles apart from you. These people are urgent, impatient and eager for action, whereas you are cautious, patient and restrained. As opposites tend to attract, Fire people will excite you with their energy and colour and they will be drawn to your quiet strength and composure. Slimming with a Fire partner could be infuriating at times. Only eat your meals with them if they are trying to slim too, or you will be constantly defending your decisions not to put butter on your vegetables or serve the fish without a pile of chips.

YOUR CREATIVE ENERGIES

If you are a typical Virgo, you tend to evaluate your days on how much you have achieved, so need outlets for your energies of the kind that produce tangible results. You usually gain more satisfaction from looking at the lawn you have carefully laid, or the sweater you knitted, than from a session of hang gliding or from walking aimlessly. There has to be a purpose for whatever you do, so start listing all the reasons you have for wanting to lose weight. .

Your taste in books probably veers towards fact, rather than fiction. Autobiographies, real life dramas, natural history, art, politics are all popular Virgo reading. Your personal collection of books probably rivals the local library, as collecting is a Virgo hobby. Miniature portraits, interesting glass bottles, unusual handicrafts, old gramophone records and brass rubbings are typical Virgo passions. One thing you cannot afford to collect, however, is fat, because it will reduce your mobility and can undermine your confidence.

Your way of unwinding is to immerse yourself in your hobbies, but you tend to do more than one thing at a time. Do you find that you write a letter and watch television at the same time, or hold an in-depth telephone conversation whilst whipping up an omelette?

Like most Virgos, you may like to travel and explore the world, scrimping and saving if necessary, to be able to afford to pay for a trip to distant parts or pastures new. Organised tours with running commentaries were designed for you as a Virgo, because you hate to miss a thing. You probably swot up on places of interest, the local history, customs and even the language of any place that you intend to visit. You cast your critical eye over the foreign vino and cuisine, taste it and pass your judgement. If you like it, it had better be low in calories, or you will return from your journey fatter than when you started it.

You are a good mixer, but are inclined to divide your time between meeting your friends and spending time on your own. Although you are not really a pace-setter, you often take responsibility in groups, for example on a committee, because you are conscientious and can be relied upon to remember the sort of details that others overlook. This exacting side of your personality helps you to succeed in home crafts and D.I.Y. projects, because you rarely leave anything to chance. This perfectionist quality is also the reason you can be certain of achieving your target weight by following your diet plan.

LIBRA

23rd SEPTEMBER TO 22nd OCTOBER

Libra is the smallest constellation in the zodiac, though it is not the least visible.

The Sun enters Libra, the sign of balance, at one of the two times of the year when the daylight hours equal the hours of darkness, (the other is in March when the Sun enters Aries) and the Libra personality constantly seeks a balance in life. This zodiac sign is ruled by Venus, which is the brightest of the planets and associated with love and harmony. Librans are rarely happy without both of these in their lives. Libra is the seventh sign of the zodiac and the cardinal (or leading) Air sign. In common with those born under the other two Air signs of Gemini and Aquarius, Libra people require enough space and freedom to follow their own interests.

YOUR SLIMMING PERSONALITY

Sometimes the Libran scales say "Ouch!" because balancing your weight with your lifestyle can be one of the most difficult juggling tricks of all for you. A balanced routine and a harmonious lifestyle are essential for you if you are to maintain a steady weight; one that doesn't keep swinging from one extreme to another according to what's happening from one week to the next.

The ancient astrologers believed that Venus ruled beauty, as well as comfort and harmony. As it is your ruling planet, it is especially important for you to have a body that pleases you when you look in your mirror. The desire to be slim and attractive is not necessarily vanity in your case, but a genuine need because you feel distressed when you know you are not looking your best. This is an excellent reason why you should start your weight loss campaign without further delay.

If you're a typical Libran, you yearn for a world that is stress-free and without pain. In fact, it is the lack of peace and tranquillity in your life that is often an underlying cause of your overweight problems, because too much aggravation or worry thoroughly upsets your equilibrium. It is by creating harmony and a beautiful world for yourself that you find fulfilment and stay healthy and in a good shape.

YOUR SLIMMING STRENGTHS

As a Libran, you're potentially an ideal candidate for a structured slimming plan (as offered in this book) because you respond well to the idea of a balanced diet, created with your personality in mind.

AIM TO PLEASE
You like to please, so treat your body in the way you treat your best friend – considerately with love and attention. Instead of treating yourself to a box of chocolates on your birthday, why not splash out on perfumed bath-fragrances or luxury body oil. The slimmer you become the longer it will last!

You will go to great lengths to look good if there is someone you wish to impress. This is one of your greatest slimming strengths, so use it to your advantage. Make a regular habit of meeting up with people who motivate you to dress up and look your best. The more often you arrange to get together with those you wish to attract, the better, because you are prepared to work hard at making sure you wont let yourself down.

You also benefit from meeting the sort of people who tend to look you up and down and judge you by your appearance. Knowing that you will be under the spotlight spurs you on to achieve your target weight. Socialise as much as possible: catching up on old school friends is always a winner because you would probably feel embarrassed to let them see you a few sizes larger than when you graduated.

One thing you can't cope with is harsh criticism, especially when you know there is something you could do to improve your size and shape. In fact, the more severe the comments you hear, the more incentive you will have to stick to your slimming plan.

In your personal book of rules for life, you believe that endeavour should always be rewarded. Equally, you don't expect to enjoy results without making an effort. The Libran symbol, the pair of delicately balanced scales, reflects the sensitivity you feel towards justice and fair play. The belief that you have that we reap what we sow happens to be a strength in regard to slimming, because you are prepared to stick to a discipline providing you know you will see a continuous weight loss.

You, above all people, also know that everything,

> **GRILL THRILL**
> Grilling grapefruit adds no calories so try it this way as a
> breakfast or main meal starter. If you consider cottage
> cheese to be uninteresting, use it as the basis for a mixed
> salad. Chop, grate or slice salad vegetables, and stir in the
> cheese. You could also add dried fruit, while cubed dry
> toast makes a delicious and scrunchy extra.

including every bar of chocolate or packet of crisps
has its price, and this awareness will be worth its
weight in gold in your daily diet plan. There is no
doubt that you have what it takes to be ruthlessly
honest with yourself and you will be the first to admit
it, if you break your diet in any way.

Fortunately, all you need to do, in the way of
atonement if you go over the top with eating, is to
sentence yourself to an extra day of dieting for the
one you gave up on. As importantly, try to analyse
the circumstances that led to your lapse, so that you
can take preventative measures in the future.

If you are true to your birth sign, you possess a
natural charm, which makes others feel at ease in
your company. No doubt you find that even
comparative strangers confide in you. This isn't
surprising because you are a wonderful listener. This
is definitely a plus factor for dieting. Once you have
heard other people's slimming-failure stories you will
be all the more keen to show that you can succeed.

Another important motivation for you to attain your
desired shape is the inner knowledge that beauty is
yours by birthright. To be slim and feel attractive is
important to your sense of worth. Constantly visualise
yourself as the shapely person you know you are

inwardly, wearing the clothes that you would like to wear, and soon will be wearing if you stick to your diet!

YOUR SLIMMING WEAKNESSES

The most difficult part of starting a new project for you is initiating the action. No-one is more expert than you at putting things off, so you are often labelled the "ditherer of the zodiac". All too often you wait for a decision to be forced upon you before you direct your energies into a new scheme or make a change. Although your intentions may be sincere, the motivation to make a start is sometimes lacking. You rarely act on impulse because you much prefer to weigh up the advantages and disadvantages of your possible course of action before making a commitment of any kind.

For you, life is about constantly striving towards finding harmony. This includes harmony of both your head and heart, as well as harmony between yourself and other people. You want to be friends with everyone, and hate to say "No", which is one of your slimming obstacles because a cross word, or a steely silence can send you scuttling to the fridge or the biscuit tin.

TREAT YOURSELF

Food is often a prime source of comfort to you, so make sure that what you eat looks good, by spending time over preparation and presentation – there's no need for diet dishes to be dull. Whether you eat from a tray or at a table, make sure it looks inviting. If you know that you're inclined to nibble when you're upset, consider non-edible forms of consolation, such as a bunch of flowers or a good book.

Another potential area of vulnerability for you is your Libran tendency to give and receive presents. It could pay you to ask your friends and family for gifts of the non-edible variety. Unwrapping a birthday present of the kind that is begging to be eaten can be disastrous, so far as your weight is concerned. You are also at risk when you are bored, with little to do, or when you are sitting still watching television or reading a book, because both situations incline you to nibble. As mentioned, Venus, the planet of comfortable living, rules your sign, so the chances are that even your first tooth was a sweet one

You are usually a good mixer because you are tactful and unassuming. When entertaining, you possess the knack of taking care of all the little touches that make your guests feel comfortable and relaxed. The food and arrangements will be presented with care and great thought. Try to put as much thought into what you are eating yourself, especially when attending or hosting a social get-together.

Be ruthless with leftovers when you entertain others. Why not provide your guests with a "doggie bag" and put the onus on them as to whether to eat up any surplus gateau or party fare?

Also, weigh up your current eating habits with those you had as a child and identify which of your food likes and dislikes are hangovers from your early years and no longer in keeping with your body's requirements.

Another slimming weakness to guard against is a tendency to bury your head in the sand if there is a problem you don't wish to face. When you need to deal with a weight problem, you cannot escape the

> **FRUIT TO SUIT**
> Eat your daily fruit allowance to suit yourself – between meals or as a starter or dessert. In fact, there doesn't have to be any set order in the way you eat. You can spread out your daily food allowance to make as many, or as few, meals as you want. Just help yourself from something on your daily list, whenever you feel like indulging in the odd snack, or treating yourself to a little something with your elevenses.

harsh fact that it's up to you to make the effort to put matters right. If you follow your diet plan on a regular basis you will eventually resolve this particular problem.

If you encounter a set-back by exceeding your permitted intake of food, it could undermine your confidence. Regard any such set-back, if one should occur, as only a temporary lapse. Simply write it off to experience and continue with your diet plan as if nothing amiss had happened.

YOU AND YOUR BODY

The theme of balance extends to your physical world, as well as your financial, social and emotional worlds. To stay slim, fit and energetic, you must balance inactive periods with time for exercise and without too much or too little of either. If you sit all day at a desk, organise action-packed sessions in the evening or at the weekends. Squash and other aggressive physical sports may be just what you need if you're deprived of physical outlets in your daily occupation. Conversely, if you're a busy housewife or spend most of the day on your feet, rushing around, opt for gentle and calming pastimes, which help you to relax and unwind. Meditation is ideal.

Your body is particularly sensitive to the wear and tear of everyday life. Subjecting yourself to too much pressure or emotional disturbance soon makes its mark on your physical being. Headaches, backaches, stomach aches and generally feeling out of sorts are usually the direct result of a conflict or an unsatisfactory situation in your work, family or love life. You are more able to stay slim and healthy when your life is ticking over quietly, than when you are involved in heavy dramas or going through periods of stress or uncertainty.

Your sign is associated with the element of Air, and it follows that fresh air is therapeutic to you. If you are to derive maximum benefit from an exercise plan, it must include opportunities to get out of doors. Don't despair, if being cooped up has caused you to pile on the pounds and expanded your vital statistics. You can usually knock yourself into shape fairly rapidly once given the right motivation. Team up with a friend or your opposite number to join an exercise or health club.

PICTURE GALLERY

Dig out your old photographs and place pictures of both the fattest and the slimmest members of your family in prominent positions in your kitchen. This will remind you in no uncertain terms of your options when you start preparing food. Don't kid yourself that you have inherited any extra inches because it's far more likely that you were conditioned, as a child, to eat larger portions than your body now needs.

The parts of your body that are particularly associated with your sign are the lumbar region (the small of the back) and the kidneys.

YOU AND YOUR EMOTIONS

Conversation is an important part of your loving. The lack of someone to talk to when you need company can drive you to the fridge for other, less healthy types of distraction: such as puddings and chocolate bars, which only create another problem for you. This is the one of being overweight. It is important that you find the courage to make the commitments called for in love because you have a great deal to offer the partner of your choice. What is more, your bathroom scales quickly reflect the state of your emotions, by showing a gain in weight whenever you feel that you're missing out on love and affection, and a weight reduction when things are going well.

As mentioned previously, the key words associated with the sign of Libra are balance and sharing, so it follows that you seek relationships that are based on mutual giving and taking. Feeling incomplete, either because you lack someone to share with, or because you are involved in an out-of-balance relationship, this may be a partnership in which you are doing most of the giving, can be very disruptive for your eating habits.

Out of all the twelve signs of the zodiac, yours is the one most likely to spend an entire life searching for your other half; your soul mate - who represents your perfect partner. That can be Libra's big mistake and cause you to miss out on the love that becomes available due to the fact that the bearer comes complete with the usual share of human failings. You rarely find complete fulfilment following a lone path in life, yet you cannot cope well with people who have overpowering or possessive personalities. As a peace-lover, you are prepared to make many allowances for those you love, so you need to be realistic about where to draw the line.

If your life partner is a fellow Libran, or born under one of the other Air signs of Gemini or Aquarius, you will have a relationship that could provide the answer to your slimming prayers, as well as your wishes in matters of the heart. A partner who is born under an Air sign will distract your thoughts from eating and be happy to spend time chatting to you whenever you feel a self-indulgent mood coming on. One thing you share with the other Air people is the ability to rationalise your own behaviour, so discussing your slimming strengths and weaknesses will help you understand yourself a little better.

Aries, Leo and Sagittarius are the three signs associated with the element of Fire. The natural bounce, energy and directness of these people will both amuse and exasperate you. You can learn a lot from their willingness to take a chance, while they will profit from watching how you carefully analyse every situation and every probability before you take the plunge. You can expect some remarkable results if you diet with a Fire person, because together you make a wonderful combination for success, especially as any excuse you make for lapsing in your diet will almost certainly be challenged.

You are often strongly attracted to those born under the Water signs. These are Cancer, Scorpio and Pisces, because their very difference appeals to you. These people judge life by what they feel and by the impressions they receive, responding instinctively to the mood of the moment, while you plan your moves and consider what you are going to say, relying on your reasoning power to guide you.

Slimming with one of the Water people could open your eyes to aspects of your eating patterns that you have failed to recognise because they will sense immediately how your food is affecting your body and they will let you know in no uncertain terms if your diet is bad news.

A relationship with a Taurus, Virgo or Capricorn, which are the three Earth signs, could prove extremely productive for you. Earth people are builders who like to have a structured plan to life. They are usually ready to work towards their goals and will also take a calculated risk if necessary. An Earth sign partner would offer you the steady support that you need and provide you with a strong shoulder to cry on in your times of troubles. At the same time, your gift of being able to look beyond the obvious will help them widen their horizons. They will also benefit from your questioning mind and flow of ideas. Even so, you could clash occasionally because Earth people seek containment, while you seek freedom. As all Earth people like to organise, they will appreciate the structure of your weight loss plan and they may even help you to sort out your meal-time arrangements.

SOME LIKE IT HOT

Hot up your main dishes with spices and herbs. You can add chilli to the mince and kidney beans, curry powder to chicken, and so on. For an eye-catching salad remember that peppers come in many shades of green, yellow and red. If you like soup, use some of your vegetable allowance for it, and try adding a shake or two of ginger or curry powder in order to ring the changes.

YOUR CREATIVE ENERGIES

Librans are well represented in the world of art and literature because yours is a very creative sign. Painting, drawing, fashion, photography, collecting beautiful pictures and possessions, these are representative of your hobbies or even your occupation. You often excel in other creative areas, such as writing and design, because you're an "ideas" person who is not unduly influenced by other people's suggestions and preferences. Make a decision to involve yourself in interests that occupy your mind whenever you feel inclined to eat out of boredom. This applies even if you prefer to observe rather than participate. All forms of dramatic display, such as the theatre, films and those activities, which feature creative expression, stimulate you and please the imaginative side of your personality.

Having personal freedom is an essential ingredient in your cake of happiness so you should plan your holidays and your spare-time activities in a way that allows you visit the wide-open spaces as much as possible. Opt for packed lunches you have prepared for yourself using part of your daily allowance, and avoid fattening but filling sausage-rolls or other savouries wrapped in pastry. Munch an apple or a carrot to allay any sudden pangs of hunger that tempts you to eat in between meals.

The sheer pleasure you derive from breathing in the pure, fresh air of the big outdoors revitalises you and helps you to cope with the demands of your everyday world. This is another contributing factor to successful dieting for you.

Your need to escape from boring routine is one of the reasons you try to pack so much into your spare time. Don't hesitate to set the pace socially or to suggest the menus when eating out, because you have what it takes to play leader to others. Even so, you are ready to let someone else take charge, providing they discuss every detail of their intentions with you before taking action. This means you can have a say when it comes to the choice of refreshments and thereby ensure that the food on offer is not damaging to your figure.

Discussion and shared interest groups are right up your street, so it can be a good idea to team up with fellow dieters. Comparing notes and progress reports will provide an extra boost to your intentions.

Not only do you take your leisure moments extremely seriously, you usually have a built in clock, which tells you when it's time for work to end and for play to begin, and vice-versa. It is when you ignore your own warning signs to ease up, or conversely to start moving, that you have problems. Your spirits then begin to dampen and your thoughts turn to food. Balance and harmony are words used so much in this chapter. This is because they are vital to your health and well-being, and they are also your personal formula for staying in shape.

SCORPIO

23rd OCTOBER TO 21st NOVEMBER

Scorpio, the eighth sign of the zodiac, is easy to spot in the heavens because it is the largest of the twelve constellations of the zodiac.

Two planets rule Scorpio: Mars, associated with energy and drive, and Pluto, the planet of power and regeneration. The Scorpio personality is powerful with strong survival instincts. Scorpio is the "fixed" (or stable) Water sign, suggesting that those born under this sign also have hidden depths and are far more sensitive than may appear on the surface. Scorpio, which is one of the earliest signs mentioned in historical records, has two symbols: The Scorpion and The Eagle. Scorpios are therefore often fiercely self-protective and security conscious, yet very ambitious.

YOUR SLIMMING PERSONALITY

Birth, death and sex are associated with your sign, so you may have noticed a distinct pattern of beginnings and endings throughout your life, representing your personal "deaths" and "rebirths". Unlike some of the other signs, who are frequently given several options at the same time, it is rare for a new door to open for you before you've closed the previous one. The way for you to slim and feel completely reborn is to turn your back completely on your old way of eating and scrap those unsatisfactory eating habits, and start afresh.

Your strong sense of self-preservation and desire to win, which make you a force to be reckoned with, can now be turned to your advantage. You can protect your health and vitality by following your diet plan. Your ability to cut your losses, rebuild and start again, even when it pains you to do so, is the perfect qualification to become a successful slimmer.

It is understandable that you wish to lose weight and look your best because Scorpio is considered to be the sexiest sign of the zodiac. Indeed, if you're a typical Scorpio, you have a natural charisma and magnetic quality, which makes others aware of your presence. You also possess the potent power to attract and hold others under your spell because they are intrigued and fascinated by you. This is all the more reason to refuse to allow your waistline to get out of control. Fortunately, your strong, resilient personality gives you the power to free yourself from those unwanted layers of surplus fat, which will give the slim, vibrant, healthy you, the opportunity to emerge.

YOUR SLIMMING STRENGTHS

Mars and Pluto, the two powerful planets, which rule your sign, are both associated with will-power and control, so it is hardly surprising that there's a part of you which has to win at all costs. Although at times this may not be to your advantage, it is a distinct point in your favour so far as slimming is concerned. Nothing is likely to stand in your way once you have set your sights on a new body-shape. You aim to be

> **LOVE FATTENS**
> Beware when the chance arises to linger over an intimate candle-lit dinner for two. Given the right companion and the right atmosphere, the food will taste better and the wine sweeter. Before you know it, you could unwittingly eat enough for both of you, as your bathroom scales will register in no uncertain terms the next day.

the boss, and usually are, so you're likely to resent food becoming more important to you than it should. Your healthy desire to rule your body with your mind, rather than allowing your appetite to be in charge, can be viewed as a valuable aid to dieting.

By controlling the amounts and the type of food that you eat, you will be able to maintain your target weight once you have achieved it!

You are tough, determined and resolute, so if you get your teeth into something, you rarely let go. When you start your slimming plan you fully expect to see it through to its completion, because you are one of those people who is unwilling to begin any project unless you seriously intend to stay with it all the way. If, by any chance, you run into problems or your plans collapse, you have what it takes to pick up the pieces and start again, and you possess the courage, the tenacity and the strength of character to do so.

You are bound to appreciate the financial benefits that come from buying smaller quantities of food. You are good at handling your cash and know how to obtain value for money by checking comparative prices and organising discounts. There's little that escapes your eagle eye and you scrutinise every detail of whatever's presented to you, working out all the implications and the possible rewards before proceeding. This means that you usually know exactly what you're letting yourself in for when you try something new and are also able to identify the particular circumstances that have led you to becoming overweight.

YOUR SLIMMING WEAKNESSES

One slimming obstacle which may have caused you to pile on the pounds, is that your eating habits usually revolve around the most recent life style you've adopted according to what you are trying to prove at any particular time and what is going on in your life. Over the years you may have switched courses more than once where food's concerned. Whether your current diet consists mainly of convenience foods from the supermarket or a health shop special, made up of a mixture of organically grown produce, ginseng and honey, it's obviously not keeping you slim, so it's time to change again. And this is one new beginning you'll be glad that you made, because a true Scorpio always likes to know that they are in peak condition.

MOOD MONITOR

Keep a record of your moods, including the way you are feeling the next time you are tempted to raid the fridge. Whether it's boredom, frustration or depression that's eating at you, write it down, and review your written analysis every week. The type of situation that threatens your peace of mind and therefore your figure, will soon become clear to you, which will enable you to come up with a solution

You can range from one extreme to another, from impressing others with your strong will, to depressing yourself with a sudden attack of self-indulgence. Life is rarely plain sailing for you, but many of the storms that can throw you off course are emotional in nature. This is because your feelings run especially deep.

> **DANGER GAMES**
> Don't neglect food awareness in your leisure moments, because you can easily become so absorbed in winning that hand of whist or Trivial Pursuits that it's not until after you've collected your prize that you realise you've eaten your way through the game without noticing.

It is your extreme sensitivity to hurt and injustice that poses your greatest slimming obstacle as you rarely forget a hurt. Like the scorpion, with a barb in its tail, which has the power to sting, you may decide to seek your revenge if someone treats you badly. Unfortunately, if you are denied the opportunity of dealing fairly and squarely with the person who has offended you, you are likely to give vent to your rage in a way that is self-destructive by eating because of anger rather than hunger.

It is not your way to give anything or anyone, including yourself, a second chance and at times, you can be altogether too inflexible. There is a stubborn, "fixed" side to your character which resists change. Be aware that this Scorpio personality trait could rob you of the success that is within your grasp

Lack of challenge or of a worthwhile motivation represents another potential threat to your figure. The feeling that your work, or your marriage or relationship, has no real direction or purpose can also cause you to attack food with a vengeance. Guard against allowing your life to become too boring or unrewarding, even if it means creating incentives for yourself at times when little is happening.

BEGIN WITH A BLITZ

Cash in on that all-or-nothing outlook on life, the hall mark of a Scorpio, by having an all out blitz on your wardrobes and drawers. You will take your mind off of the food cupboards if you use your spare time to sort out your clothes - with an eye to keeping what you will still be able to wear when you no longer need to diet.

Another potential slimming obstacle is your readiness to drive yourself on relentlessly, which can cause you to take drastic measures if you suddenly decide that you want to lose half a stone rapidly. It's possible you've tried to shed surplus pounds in the past by trying "crash" or extreme diet methods you may have even fasted. As you discovered, these tactics always fail in the end. As you know, you are not a person who is easily impressed or influenced, which in some ways is commendable. But be careful that you are not denying yourself the chance of profiting from other people's knowledge and experience.

Your independent nature inclines you to be unwilling to confide all of your thoughts. This means that you often struggle alone with problems unnecessarily, when help and advice is available. The specialist information already amassed in your weight loss plan makes it possible for you to diet safely and comfortably, knowing that you will ultimately measure up to your ideal size. The decision to follow my star guide to losing weight is one you will be glad you made.

YOU AND YOUR BODY

The reproductive organs and the pelvis are the parts of the body ruled by Scorpio. That is why your sign is linked with regeneration, sex and also the birth and death of the species. Your ability to regenerate your own body stands you in good stead if ever your health is under par. You manage to draw on supplies of inner strength which help you fight off many of the everyday ailments to which some of your peers succumb. Maintaining a sensible weight for your size and knowing your appearance doesn't let you down is important for your self-esteem. Your body, health and eating patterns are strongly influenced by your moods and the state of your mind. Therefore, your forceful energy needs to be channelled correctly for you to stay on top form. You can suffer from extremes of weight if you lack motivation and a challenge of one kind or another. It pays you to include regular energetic physical exercise in your daily programme. Those Scorpios who are sports orientated will gravitate towards competitive games because the chance to win while you're letting off steam suits your determined personality. You may be attracted to one or more of the martial arts, such as judo or karate.

SECRET MISSION

In your heart, you may wish to keep your diet a secret. Therefore, it's as well that your diet plan requires you to give just one week over to serious slimming at a time, and it also allows for packed lunches. No one needs to know your intentions until the pounds have slipped away and your new measurements and improved shape are being noticed and admired.

However, if you loathe sport or contrived exercise, you'll be happy to know that digging the garden, a lively spate of housework, or polishing the car, will serve equally well to tone you up and keep you in shape, by burning up some of your excess calories and energy. There is no need to punish your body in your fight against your flab: walking briskly or swimming represent excellent, alternative forms of exercise. Touch and body contact mean a lot to you as a sensual Scorpio, so you'll especially benefit from a soothing massage whenever you feel tense or need to unwind. An ideal massage for you is the type used in aromatherapy, where essential oils are matched to your particular personality type. If your budget doesn't run to a professional treatment don't despair. You can do yourself a power of good by smoothing on a body-balm, all over, to relax your muscles gently after a hot shower or bath. Treating your skin to loving care, from day one of your diet, will help avoid stretch marks appearing as your store cupboard of fatty flesh gradually disappears.

As Scorpio is a Water sign, you should regard water as the liquid that nature intends you to drink. Not only does it add to that full-up feeling, it is non-fattening, inexpensive and cleanses and purifies your system. Why not pour out a glass of the fizzy mineral sort for yourself and sip it before and in-between your meals?

YOU AND YOUR EMOTIONS

Although Scorpio is a sign associated with sex, many Scorpios stay unmarried. The fear of making a mistake and being hurt can be even stronger than the passions that burn up inside you. If only your fat cells would burn up in the same way! You seek written guarantees in love because you need to know that your chosen one will have eyes only for you and be faithful to you forever. If they're not, you're sure to find out because you possess an uncanny knack of being able to detect the truth, as others learn to their cost if they try to cover up their actions with lies or excuses. You even manage to ferret out things you're not supposed to know. Just to be totally infuriating, you somehow manage to keep your own secrets carefully hidden.

You possess a powerful capacity to love and protect those you care about. You are passionate, loyal and a person of commitment. You need to feel very close to your partner in a relationship. Ideally they must be ready to take your ambitions seriously, as well as your talents, priorities and, most importantly, your principles. Apart from all this they must be as self-motivated as you are because if there's one thing you can't abide, it's someone you consider to be weak and spineless. Even with this short shopping list in the love department, you can begin to understand why some of your fellow Scorpios stay single, often travelling a lonely road in life, not realising that they have passed by more than one potentially suitable partner in their endless search for perfection.

Whether or not you are happily matched, be aware that demanding too much from another human being and refusing to accept their failings can only result in disenchantment, which can be one of the root causes of overweight problems for you.

Once you've accepted the initial differences between you and an Aries, Leo or Sagittarius, these are the Fire sign people (their lack of subtlety when they want something, and their different emotional needs), you'll discover that there are many similarities. Like you they are fairly dynamic and ambitious, as well as self-motivated. The spirit of adventure that burns within all Fire people is attractive to you and so is their ability to look on the bright side of life. One of the things that they like about you is that you're a challenge. It can take them forever to figure you out, that is, if they ever do. A Fire sign partner or friend makes an ideal slimming companion for you because their eagerness to see results, which will make them persist in their dieting, come what may, is the encouragement you need to prove that you're also a winner.

A relationship with a person born under one of the three Earth signs, Taurus, Virgo or Capricorn, could satisfy many of your needs, because like you, they are security conscious and work to a plan of campaign. However, Earth people regard food as one of the prime sources of security, so tend to offer edible gifts for anniversaries and as tokens of their appreciation. Even so, they respond positively to logic and common-sense, so your Earth companions will be supportive to your slimming efforts if you point out the numerous benefits you and they, if applicable, can gain from losing weight.

There is a natural flow between you and other Water people, Scorpios, like yourself or Cancer or Pisces. They will soothe you when you feel stressed, comfort you in times of trouble and help you relax. You will feel comfortable and at ease in the presence of a Water friend or partner because you are both sensitive and intuitive. This means that you stand a good chance of enjoying wedded bliss together, especially as you both seek permanency in a relationship. Your mutual empathy can be of great value in a joint weight reduction effort because you will sense when each other is in the mood to nibble and know the precise preventative measures to take for the circumstances, as well as what to say to each other in order to boost each other's morale if the bathroom scales suddenly register disappointment.

Those born under the three Air signs of Gemini, Libra and Aquarius deal with life's problems in a entirely different way to you. They are thinkers, who analyse and question everything, including their own emotions. They are firm believers in mind over matter and brain cells over fat cells. They are often at odds with themselves and their passions and feelings tend to be suppressed, or regarded as irrational. If you team up with one of these people you will make an unlikely couple, but it can work out if you find a common cause and allow each other to have a certain amount of personal space and independence. Even so, you would have to curb your Scorpio possessiveness, as all Air people need to be able to flit away on their own occasionally, without being asked too many questions.

YOUR CREATIVE ENERGIES

Scorpios are known for their nose for a mystery and ability to investigate and find what is hidden. This gift may draw you to hobbies, which involve a degree of research or detective work. Collecting antiques and archaeology are classic Scorpio type interests. You also adore a competition or a puzzle and may play cards, chess, dominos or other competitive games.

SECRET WEAPONS

When it comes to fashion, your sign and style is associated with all that is downright sexy. Which is why you should refuse to become a frump by trying to conceal surplus pounds under drab, or dowdy clothes. Dress smart, and while you work away at whittling down your waist line, plan the sort of outfit you will buy, which should be one that will knock them cold, once you have reached your target weight.

Discovery holidays were made for you because they provide the means to roll a challenge and an adventure into one glorious experience. Wherever you go, you need to explore and satisfy yourself that you have seen all there is to see and you tend to notice what less observant signs have overlooked.

You love music in all its forms and may also be passionate about the arts and literature. You expect to spend a lot of your leisure time on your own, but it is good for you to choose a few spare-time activities that you can share with others. You are a good listener and can also make a valuable contribution to any debate.

Your social style leans towards intimate get-togethers, especially twosomes or rendezvous with a few tried and tested friends. While you will attend or give a large party if there's a good reason to do so, you are happiest in the cosy companionship of a small group. When it's your turn to entertain others, you do so, like so much of your life, with careful thought and planning. This means you can follow your diet allowances without any real problems. It is when the boot's on the other foot and someone's is entertaining and wining and dining you, that you must be on your guard.

You can be a dedicated 'do-it-yourselfer', ready to tackle anything, from hanging wallpaper to laying a parquet floor. You prefer to have a purpose and a goal in sight when you allocate your time and energy to a spare-time activity. You soon get stuck in to your latest enthusiasm, once you are sure of what is required. This will help you make a positive start to your diet and exercise regime. Renovation is your forte, whether that's a modest touch of 'make-do-and-mend' or something more ambitious, such as rebuilding an engine or restoring a priceless work of art. As you are rarely daunted, you may take pleasure in tackling projects that others consider impossible. This means that no matter how much weight you have to shift, you' can do it! You are capable and enjoy pitting your wits against a problem.

Never forget that the sign of Scorpio is associated with birth and death and one of the most powerful signs in the zodiac. The regenerative forces that flow through you will help you let old ways of life die and new ones begin, so that you can enjoy every day in the best of health, knowing you look as good as you feel.

SAGITTARIUS

22nd NOVEMBER TO 21st DECEMBER

The constellation of Sagittarius, which is the ninth sign of the zodiac and a fire sign, is symbolised by the mythological Centaur – half man and half beast, representing the struggle between the baser instincts of Man and the aspirations of the higher self. The typical Sagittarius personality is restless, enterprising and eager to learn all that there is to learn in life. By tradition, the Centaur holds a bow and arrow, which is why Sagittarius is also called the sign of the Archer.

Mighty Jupiter, the largest of the planets recognised in astrology as well as in our universe, rules Sagittarius. It's journey through the zodiac takes approximately twelve years. This tends to be reflected in the lives of Sagittarius people, with important changes occurring every twelve years. Jupiter is the planet of expansion and associated with good fortune. Sagittarians usually have a strong faith in their own good luck, which is often justified because of their ability to think positively and thereby attract the ways and means to make their dreams come true.

YOUR SLIMMING PERSONALITY

As a Sagittarian, you make a very good dieting subject

because your eternal optimism makes you confident that you will succeed. Your expansive attitudes extend to all areas of your life, which you intend to live to the full. You are likely to set your sights high with regard to losing weight. However, it is only too easy for those ruled by Jupiter, which as mentioned relates to the principle of expansion, to do so literally and increase their vital statistics due to gaining weight as the years pass by.

You firmly believe in tomorrow but must guard against under-valuing that which is readily available or happening in the present. As a perpetual schemer and planner, one who is ready to make changes and take chances, you will have to accept that retaining a weight loss is only possible by eating wisely on a daily basis. You, in particular, must make healthy eating the rule rather than the exception.

YOUR SLIMMING STRENGTHS

In many respects you are a born gambler because you are naturally adventurous and ready to try most things at least once. You will be happy to be the first one in your circle of friends and acquaintances to try the star guide way of losing weight. You can throw yourself into a new project with a speed and a confidence that leaves others standing. This self-assurance and eagerness to see tangible results represents an important slimming strength and it will help you to achieve your target weight.

Like the other two Fire signs, which are Aries and Leo, you possess energy and enthusiasm, which is directed in whatever you do. The shopping, the cooking, the measuring out of controlled portions,

TROLLEY TEMPTATIONS

Instead of racing around the supermarket with a laden trolley, scooping up panic buys of convenience food (due to that impulsive invitation you gave to friends or neighbours "to come around to my place for a bite to eat") take your time to write a carefully thought out list and pay special attention to calorie values.

you will take all of these in your stride. The supermarket will become a whole new world to you.

You love to learn and also to share what you learn with others. This has earned you the reputation of being the teacher of the zodiac. Once you have proof that your diet really works, you will be anxious to share the secret of your success with your overweight friends or family. You're unlikely to be considered a diet bore because your sense of humour and amusing way of telling a tale will make others eager to listen to your slimming stories. It will not take much persuasion on your part to convince them that they should follow your lead. Another advantage of talking about your weight-reducing plan is that it will strengthen your conviction that it's the right way of life for you to follow as well.

If you are a typical Sagittarian, you are at your happiest when planning for the future. You possess a breadth of vision, which enables you to identify your next main objective and "go for it". This ability to visualise and believe in tomorrow is another valuable slimming strength; one that will assist your battle with overweight. Imagine yourself the shape and the size that you would like to be because, once you have done this you will be half way there!

FIT FOR ANYTHING

Try to exercise every day, even if it means having to snatch a few minutes here and a few minutes there. The motto for you is NEVER put off until tomorrow the press-ups or brisk walk that matters today. An exercise bike or a rowing machine will help you to fight the flab and also keep your circulation toned up, no matter what the weather is doing outside.

Once you rise to a challenge, you are not easily discouraged. Indeed, it's probably true to say that a challenge brings out the best in you because you certainly enjoy proving that you can succeed. Few put in as much effort as you do, once you are fired with an ambition. Make your next ambition one that will benefit you in more ways than one. This is to lose weight and wear the clothes that make you feel good about yourself.

There is an honesty and frankness about your personality that can both please and offend other people. You are unlikely to bat an eyelid when telling your host or hostess that their chocolate gateau is "for fatties only". Fortunately, you usually manage to make people laugh when you are outspoken, so are quickly forgiven. This forthrightness is an asset in your fight against flab because you will not be reluctant to request a substitute when faced with a figure threatening dessert.

YOUR SLIMMING WEAKNESSES

One of the obstacles that faces many Sagittarians is the fact that they are impulsive eaters and react instantly when a pang of hunger strikes. This may result in eating cream cakes, chocolate bars, nuts, crisps and the sort of snacks that are appetising but laden with calories. The same applies to what you drink, because many brands of wine, beer and refreshing bottles of fizz contain large quantities of sugar, which, in turn, converts to unwanted fat.

Make a point of differentiating between need and desire when you reach for a handy snack and take a firm line with yourself if you realise that boredom is the true motivation for any tendency to nibble in between meals.

Your gregarious nature and generosity probably prompts you to urge your friends to have one last helping of food or a last drink, when offering them hospitality. The chances are you follow suit, which can be bad news for your diet.

Another potential weight loss obstacle is impatience, which can cause you to abandon a scheme before it has been given a fair trial. By the same token, it can also incline you to roar ahead too quickly for your own good. It's essential to follow the weight loss plan as prescribed if you hope to reach your target weight and prevent the fat from returning overnight.

One of your innermost yearnings is likely to be associated with being able to travel. Ideally, you

ABROAD VIEW
In many countries, you only have to look around and study the shape of the native population to establish that their traditional fare, as tempting as it is, is very fattening. Satisfy your taste for the unusual by rationing experimental eating to delicious foreign fruits and crunchy local salads – without using too much oil.

should be free to pack a suitcase at a moment's notice and spread your wings, even if just for a weekend away with friends. You love to explore the world and see new places, new faces and at the same time sample new foods. Sadly, this doesn't always go hand in hand with watching your weight. When you are away from your home, do your best to be diet-conscious. Curb your penchant for interesting looking dishes of the kind that are loaded with fat, as well as flavour. Play safe and opt for grilled food, salads and fresh vegetables.

The average shape of the local population should provide you with an insight into the fattening potential of the traditional fare so bear this in mind as you consider the merits of 'the dish of the day'.

YOU AND YOUR BODY

The hips, bottom and thighs are the parts of the body ruled by Sagittarius. It is to your distinct advantage to give due consideration to your own because they are likely to provide a clear indication of the times in the future when you should return to you're your weight loss plan. Take note, and do something about it immediately if you suddenly realise that you've gained an extra helping of wobbly fat on your bottom or tops of your legs.

Your remarkable capacity to enjoy life means that your weight problems, as well as any feelings of being 'run down' can sometimes be linked with boredom, or the lack of a worthwhile goal or interest. It is to your own advantage to take whatever steps are needed to ensure that your existence never becomes too humdrum or uneventful.

As the adventurer of the zodiac, you seek constant

FUEL FOR THOUGHT
Invest as much careful thought into the choice of fuel for your body as you normally put to the fuel you buy for your car, and be prepared to change the habits of a lifetime by offloading your store of chocolate bars and savoury nibbles. It's pointless knowing that you're really a lively, sleek, racing model if other people look at you and think that you're built like a tank!

stimulus and excitement, and should try to be out and about as much as possible, exploring new activities and broadening your horizons generally. The great outdoors represents the perfect exercise ground for you, whether you're sporting a bat and ball or jogging in the park. Camping, walking, ball games or boating, all will keep the roses in your cheeks, your mind off food and act like a tonic for your health. The community sports centre is also ideal Sagittarian territory. Sitting moping in front of the television for long periods is definitely bad news for you.

However, the frantic pace of your life can sometimes leave you depleted, and it may not be until you feel utterly exhausted, that you take the time to sit back and take stock of your body – only to find that it is has begun to look neglected or is very much the worse for wear. Bear in mind that, no matter how active you like to be you are not super human and like everyone else, you need to relax at times and ease out of the fast lane. Otherwise tension is likely to build up and take its toll on your neck, back and shoulders. Frustration and anxiety are other potential enemies to your well being, as well as to your figure and weight.

SNAP HAPPY
Use that new digital camera to take a photograph of yourself now, bulges and all, and then taken another one in a week's time and so on, to supply pictorial evidence of how you're doing. As they say, "the camera never lies", so your photos will make it clear to you when you've achieved your ideal weight. With the help of your weight loss plan you will be able to stay that way.

YOU AND YOUR EMOTIONS

There's a very sensitive, romantic person hiding behind that breezy exterior. If you're true to your sign you are something of a dreamer, an incurable idealist, and a total softy at heart. Companionship is an essential part of a close relationship to you, so your partner must also be your very best friend. Warm, affectionate and energetic, you need to be with someone who shares your sense of adventure and is equally independent. They must also accept your restlessness and desire to be your own person. Most importantly, they must know how to let their hair down and have fun, as the ability to laugh and enjoy life together, and even slim together, is the only successful recipe for you where affairs of the heart are concerned.

However, you can become dissatisfied once you are in the position to be able to take love for granted. What is more, your endless search for excitement can be the root cause of emotional upsets and arguments. Try to come to terms with your constant desire for action and do your best to keep the path of true love running smoothly. Fortunately, you won't become restless, bored or inclined to stray from your weight loss plan, which has been designed with your active type of personality in mind.

Your sunny, outgoing disposition attracts others instantly. It doesn't take long for your friendly approach and sense of humour to break down barriers, even of those who are stuffy or reserved. Other people fascinate you and you are prepared to go out of your way to meet anyone who sounds interesting. You love to cheer people up and offer them encouragement if they feel depressed. One of the fringe benefits of achieving your own target weight will be the positive impression it will make on the friends you have who are unhappily overweight.

Some may look at you and assume that you haven't a care in the world because you rarely confide your deepest feelings to anyone, not even the one who knows you best. You'll be the first to crack a joke about your diet intentions but deep down, you're well aware of the serious reasons behind your need to get to grips with your surplus weight. You know, instinctively, that fat slows you down. **The truth is it not only looks unsightly, it can also put a strain on your heart.**

A relationship with someone born under a Fire sign; a Sagittarian like yourself or a Leo or Aries, should prove stimulating for the both of you. They share your hankering to be at the centre of the action. You can both be extravagant and are also likely to challenge each other but they will be able to handle your directness and occasional lack of subtlety. They may even appreciate the fact that they will always know where they stand with you. You view life in the same way as they do, with the belief that everything you want will be yours eventually. As a slimming companion, you couldn't do better, because both of you are willing to go after what you want. This double helping of determination is enough to ensure that together you'll achieve your targets.

It's a completely different story when it comes to you and a Water sign person. These are the signs of Cancer, Scorpio or Pisces. Water sign people are highly sensitive and emotional, with a tendency to take things personally. If you pass a light-hearted comment of the kind that could be interpreted as a criticism, when you see your Water sign colleague or spouse diving into a bag of sweets or crisps, you are likely to provoke an angry response or even worse, a hurt silence.

Nevertheless, you have a great deal to offer each other, but must take one or two important differences into consideration. You may find it hard to cope with a Water sign person's constant need for reassurance, while they can feel threatened by your impulsiveness and quick temper. On a positive note, they will calm you down when you feel stressed and they will listen to your problems and help you put them into perspective. They will offer support and backing even if it means putting themselves out for you. In return, you would be a good friend for an overweight Water sign individual because your gift of being able to tell others what's good for them will soon have them sold on the idea that need to stay with their diet.

Expect to have a good rapport with someone born under one of the three Air signs. These are Gemini, Libra and Aquarius. Although Air sign people possess an air of coolness and detachment about them, while you, as a Fire person, come across as warm and enthusiastic, you have what it takes to make a good combination. They will appreciate your fiery strengths, while you will adore their ability to talk about this, that and everything. You stand to benefit from joining forces with an Air sign person when following your weight loss plan because they are objective and will not hesitate to analyse any lapse on your part and give you the reasons why you failed to stick to your diet. This will enable you to take preventative measures so that it doesn't happen again.

An Earth sign person, a Taurus, Virgo or Capricorn, could add a degree of security to your life. The very nature of Earth sign people is to seek lasting situations, to stabilise and put down roots. Your bold approach to life and willingness to take a risk, if the occasion demands it, will encourage an Earth sign partner to make the most of their own opportunities. At the same time, your drive and positive manner will provide the necessary boost for them to slim. They will find it hard to comprehend your desire to explore and experiment, but they will be realistic enough to

---

WATCH OUT!

Be aware of what is really in a drink when you dine out or socialise. Alcohol and fizzy drinks add calories without nutrients. They also stimulate your appetite. Alcohol, in particular, does this and also manages to dull your senses, so that your resolve weakens. Limit your drinks and you will keep a clear head, which will be good news the next morning. You will also have the satisfaction of knowing that you completed another day of your weight loss plan successfully.

accept that that's the way you are. Meanwhile, you can learn from their structured way of dealing with problems and find out where you should slow down. An Earth partner will encourage you to stick to your diet plan and also to eat your weight loss meals in the correct order and one day's ration at a time!

YOUR CREATIVE ENERGIES

You probably love speed. Do you remember as a child wanting to shoot ahead on your bicycle or skate board and be faster than everyone else? As an adult you may still hanker after a fast car so you can zoom off into the sunset whenever the mood grabs you. This risk-taking element within you, the part of you that quite enjoys dancing with danger, is your creative force, surging up within you searching for an outlet. Unfortunately, a weight reducing plan is one thing that shouldn't be hurried, so you now need patience and perseverance, two qualities that rarely come naturally to those born under your sign.

Whether you are young or old, you probably possess a great zest for life and desire to involve yourself in all sorts of activities. You are versatile and ready to have a go at anything, and you may even be multi-talented. The shadow side of this image is seen in the Sagittarians who are over-optimistic about their ability to deliver and so disperse their energies in many different directions, which means they fail to become proficient in anything. Learning to invest your time carefully is the most certain way for you to find success, so don't stray from your diet plan. This is one occasion when you should make up your mind to stay totally single minded.

Sagittarius people are often entertaining story-tellers and make excellent show-biz personalities or scintillating sales-people because they excel in front of an audience. This trait can assist you now, especially if you need to encourage others to help you with your weight loss plan. Enthusing your friends and loved ones with your ideas and expectations will serve to reinforce your own intentions.

You pour a great deal of creative energy into your social life and can usually come up with a bright idea on where to go for an outing. Your personality thrives on any kind of group activity, and you understand the true party spirit and want others to enjoy themselves as much as you do. If at all possible, you should join up with friends who are also on weight reducing diets and eat together. In the process, you can swap humorous dieting experiences and progress reports.

CAPRICORN

22nd DECEMBER TO 19th JANUARY

Although the constellation of Capricorn, the tenth sign of the zodiac, is not especially easy to locate in the heavens, it was regarded by the ancient astrologers to be a very sacred sign, because it governs the period in the Northern hemisphere, when the days start to grow longer and the hours of darkness begin to lessen.

Ruled by the slow moving planet Saturn, a planet associated with structure, those born under Capricorn are considered to be patient, careful, self controlled and ambitious. The sure-footed Goat, able to climb to the top of the highest mountain, symbolises this sign, which is a sign of leadership and the tenth in the zodiac. The Capricorn individual is concerned with tradition and possesses a strong urge to instil order into their surroundings.

YOUR SLIMMING PERSONALITY

Capricorn is considered to be the sign of the establishment and associated with government, law and order, so it is natural for you to seek a set of rules for your life. In fact, when you were a child, you may have been especially conscientious. When you think back, do you remember being put in charge of your brothers or sisters, or friends in order to keep an eye on what they were doing? The answer to this is almost certainly "yes", because even little Capricorns tend to possess an air of authority and ability to take control. As an adult, you are likely to feel happiest when there are recognisable guide-lines to follow, which makes you a superb candidate for an organised slimming programme. The written instructions, the carefully planned diets and the do's and the don'ts, are exactly the style of language that any law-abiding Capricorn appreciates.

Capricorns are reputed to be the planners and builders of the zodiac, and many Capricorns go right to the top of their chosen occupations. It is a mistake for others to assume you are unadventurous or afraid of change, because this is not the case at all. However, you prefer to think things through thoroughly before making firm decisions. You look to the future but also value tradition and the past. Once you have done your homework and made a decision, you can leave others standing because like the Goat, (usually a nifty mover) which symbolises your sign, you have what it takes to make fast progress and arrive at your chosen destination safely. You now have the chance to be both nimble and agile, which is the perfect motivation to be able to stick to your weight loss plan, especially if you have realised that too much weight is beginning too slow you down.

YOUR SLIMMING STRENGTHS
Whether you are male or female, bear in mind that the Capricorn image is elegant and sophisticated. Your awareness of how you should look is a plus factor for

GRAPPLING WITH GREENS

The Earth sign diet allows unlimited quantities of salads and green vegetables. The ball is in your court to make them interesting, which is where your fertile imagination comes into its own. Eat Spinach, Broccoli, Brussel Sprouts, French Beans, Peas and Lettuce and also experiment with any produce that is new in your experience.

your slimming ambitions. The mere thought of being described as a "corpulent Capricorn" should motivate you to set your sights high and persevere with your weight loss plan, until the day that your tape measure gives its approval.

Your ambitious streak tends to drive you on until you have achieved exactly what you have set out to do. You are willing to accept responsibility and will even practice self-denial if it will assist in the pursuit of your objectives. A gift for quiet concentration and a readiness to do the groundwork before making a new beginning also indicates that you will be a winner in the slimming stakes. In fact, you already have the ideal weapons to assure victory in the fight against flab.

A gift that most Capricorns possess is an uncanny sense of timing. This provides you with an edge on your competitors in games or pastimes that depend on precision, such as football, netball, rugby and hockey. You also appreciate the need to abide by the rules, which is a plus point when it comes to sticking to your weight loss plan.

Did you know that it is important to keep your survival mechanism under control to slim successfully? The way to do this is to eat slightly less than your

FORGIVE YOURSELF

Capricorns can be unrelenting taskmasters, making life hard for themselves as well as others. However, if your resolve weakens, which it could do on occasion seeing as you're only human – be ready to forgive yourself. Just continue with your weight loss plan the following day as if nothing amiss has happened.

daily calorific requirements, without cutting back on the essential vitamins, mineral salts and other nutrients that your body needs to be efficient. At the same time, you should step up your physical activities, which will help burn up the excess fat that you want to lose. In this way you will rev up your metabolism and your weight will start to lessen accordingly. Crash diets never work because they cause ravenous hunger and tiredness and slow down the functions of the body.

Your determination is another of your slimming strengths. What is more, in common with the signs of Taurus and Virgo, you possess a "down to earth" quality, which helps you to keep your feet on the ground and do the right thing if you are put in a situation that is challenging. This will be invaluable if you are bombarded with temptations of the edible variety.

It has taken you a long time, possibly years, to reach your present weight, so if you try to slim too quickly, expect your body to put up strong resistance. Losing weight gradually ensures that the pounds lost aren't regained the moment you ease up a little. Fortunately, you are not one to be impressed by promises of quick and spectacular weight losses. It was probably a Capricorn who first said that "if it's worth having, it's worth waiting for" because you are realistic as well as patient. This patience is a wonderful Capricorn slimming strength, because it will enable you to reduce your size at a steady and sensible speed, and make good progress without finding that you have depleted your energies

Money also comes into the equation because the savings you will be able to make when you start to buy less food, will appeal to you. Your appreciation of the many possible uses of money, especially your own, will help you to resist buying food items on impulse when they are surplus to the requirements of your weight loss plan.

YOUR SLIMMING WEAKNESSES

Conservation is a key factor in your life because the evolved Capricorn protects and preserves the inherited resources and traditions of society. You may be interested in restoring old buildings or act as a leading light in the ecology movement. Even if you're not, it's likely that you place great store in the customs you've grown up with, and refuse to make any change purely for the sake of it. This represents your greatest

---

ALERT TO DANGER

Learn awareness eating, which means no nibbling while concentrating on something other than food. In the past the weight could have been creeping on without you noticing it. Perhaps because you were munching away while you were reading or watching television. Make it a rule to always set a table or tray and sit down while you concentrate on your meal and then your brain will register that you've eaten your fill.

slimming obstacle, because it is your previous life style that has padded you out and therefore, you may have to close the door on some of your past eating patterns once you follow the weight loss plan that is right for your star sign group. The fact that you are concerned about your weight indicates that the time has come to adopt a new lifestyle based on present knowledge about the workings of the body and metabolism, and how fat is stored.

You possess an excellent sense of timing, but this can be a two-edged sword when it comes to slimming, especially if you are in the habit of taking frequent breaks for refreshments. Your body-clock will continue to ring its alarm bells, to tell you it's time for tea and toast, or coffee and cakes, unless you reset it to a different timetable. This is one that will fit in with a weight conscious style of eating. Munch on a stick of celery or a small apple to appease any unsatisfied appetite you have in the early days of dieting. It will not be long before you will be able to do without eating snacks in-between meals.

Another potential slimming hazard for you is the

TRICK AND TREAT

Here's another trick of the slimming trade, one to give you a head start in the war against weight-gain. Pile your plate up with food that is low in calories, and you will feel as if you are eating twice as much. A little food will go a long way with the help of a few kitchen gadgets. Set your slicing machine on THIN for cucumber, onions or potatoes and use a fine grater for cheese or carrot. Follow this method and two spoonfuls will turn into a satisfying-looking mound of appetising food.

Saturnine or "heavy", serious side to the Capricorn personality. This can sometimes incline you to look on the gloomy side of life and impose unnecessary limitations on yourself. Feeling low or dispirited can act like a brake on your diet, and cause your will-power to weaken. A deep-rooted Capricorn idea, that needs examining, is the conviction that you were fated to carry a heavy load in life because this is what you're doing literally at present, in the form of the fat distributed in generous layers around your body.

Many Capricorns suffer from such a lack of confidence when young that they wait until the second part of their lives to realise the dreams of youth. Whatever your age, don't stand in your own path now, especially as it's highly probable that you have been the one to encourage others to succeed in previous projects related to self-improvement. Follow your own sensible advice to resolve your overweight problem and make your next assignment one that improves your figure.

Guard against trying to compensate for an aching heart, a disappointment or simply a feeling of being "down", with a pick-me-up in the shape of a box of chocolates or packet of savouries. The moment you sense that an attack of the proverbial 'blues' could strike, immerse yourself interests of the sort that are guaranteed to cheer you up and provide non fattening pleasure.

YOU AND YOUR BODY

If you're a typical Capricorn, you are keenly interested in the workings of your body, so are ready to take positive action to put matters right if you become aware, or even faintly suspicious, that all is not well. The second part of a Capricorn's life is usually when the snuffles, coughs and chills that plague them in childhood, teens and twenties, are firmly behind them. Whether you are enjoying the first flush of youth or looking forward to retirement, you will appreciate the need to stay healthy and in good shape to enjoy the full benefits that you, as a Capricorn, can derive with maturity.

Your bones, especially your knees, are the parts of your anatomy ruled by Capricorn, so make a point of doing exercises that will keep you supple, as part of a daily limbering-up routine. Yours is a fairly physical sign, so regular keep fit sessions should become as much of a habit as brushing your teeth. However, gently does it at first.

Your body will also benefit from another healthy habit, one that is low in cost and especially relevant if you're a "night owl". This is to refrain from eating your main meal very late at night because it takes longer to burn calories up once you've "switched off" and gone to sleep. Food eaten immediately prior

---

LOG THE LOSSES

Why not start a 'slimming journal' that will be an inspiration to your children in the future. Make a weekly note of your weight and comment on the way it varies between the 'two weeks of strict dieting' and the 'four weeks of moderation' that comprise your Earth sign diet. Remember to add dates and prices of food, where you shopped and any other relevant facts. You could even mention the weather and your mood from day to day. You will be creating your own piece of history.

to bed-time stands far more chance of being filed away as fat. It may interest you to know that you use only about 30 calories an hour once you are asleep. This is the amount of calories supplied by one very small apple.

Laughter is a great tonic and a powerful preventative medicine against illness, as well as a boost for you as a potential slimmer. Being over-concerned with the worries of the world and other people's problems, as well as your own, can weigh you down and depress you. It can also drive you to find consolation of the edible kind! You may still be carrying the evidence of your last bout of worrying around your waistline.

You probably prefer to follow set patterns of eating and drinking. At this point it is to your advantage to reconsider your ideas about food. This is especially relevant if you are a member of an overweight family. Your excess pounds are more likely to be the effects of overloading your plate for years than due to glandular reasons. It's to your advantage to become used to your correct diet plan well before your next family reunion.

YOU AND YOUR EMOTIONS

It is likely that there are certain similarities between your approach to affairs of the heart and your approach to slimming because you are deliberate and realistic about your emotional needs. Although hearts and flowers are not necessarily your style, you seek a deep and meaningful emotional relationship and regard marriage or a long-term commitment, as a natural development. You rarely give your heart completely unless there's a contract for life offered in return. It doesn't take you long to make up your mind when you meet someone who is a potential partner, even if you choose to keep them guessing or at arm's length for a while. Having a clear structure or framework is as important to you in your love-life as in your diet and fitness plan, because you like to know the rules, the chances of success and the possible future developments, in whatever you do.

Ideally your partner should share your long-term ambitions, as well as your practical approach to life. They should also be reliable, resourceful and wildly exciting! He or she needs to appreciate and bring out your delightful sense of humour, which is sometimes lost on those who lack subtlety. You can be wonderfully romantic, in fact more romantic than some would believe possible. Underneath that self-disciplined and sensible exterior, there's a passionate heart ticking away, but the defensive barrier you put up if you're uncertain of someone's intentions can make you appear cool, even icy and indifferent. You tend to be a self-contained person, but don't miss out on the encouragement and support available from friends and loved ones, who may even like to diet along with you.

You relate well to those born under the Water signs of Cancer, Scorpio and Pisces, Once a Water sign friend or relative decides to help you slim, they will do everything in their power to help you, even if that means eating stringently themselves, in order to stop you feeling that you're missing out. However, as caring and loving as your Water sign companions are, don't accept their hospitality unless they have been told you're following a diet because their basic urge is to feed and look after others. Even so, this is a non-competitive and mutually supportive combination, which will work well in both business and emotional relationships.

The people born under the Fire signs of Aries, Leo and Sagittarius, can add an element of excitement to life. However, their liking for action and desire to proceed at a fast pace may prove taxing for your nerves and composure. The Fire sign personality is usually fairly assertive but doesn't always appreciate that what's right for them, may not be right for others. Despite this, a Fire sign partner makes a wonderful slimming ally because even without speaking, they will make you feel incredibly guilty, just by the way that they look at you, whenever you reach for that biscuit tin or an extra helping of dinner.

The Air sign people, Gemini, Libra and Aquarians, are always receptive to the winds of change, so if you hope to tempt an Air sign partner into joining you in your weight loss campaign, sell them the thought that you are ready to give a new way of eating a try. A long-term partnership with an Air sign person requires a great deal of effort and understanding on both sides because while you prefer to see one project through at a time, in the Air sign person's book it is quite O.K. to change direction at a moment's notice.

WINNING COMBINATIONS
Cook a combination of meat, poultry, or fish with vegetables, water and herbs and make a casserole. You can now buy low-fat portions of meat and poultry. You can also add a small quantity of low-fat spread to a baked potato if you're drooling for butter.

Life with one of the Earth sign people, a Taurus, Virgo or fellow Capricorn, will be fairly predictable and well organised. You will find many things to agree about so this relationship can work, providing you are allowed to make your own decisions. Bear in mind that as the cardinal Earth sign you are a leader and are unlikely to find true fulfilment with anyone who constantly questions your actions. An Earth sign companion will share your methodical approach to problems, so you will be able to back each other up with dozens of practical reasons for losing weight, if either one of you starts to waiver. Where slimming is concerned, this should prove a successful combination

YOUR CREATIVE ENERGIES

Many fine musicians, potters, sculptors, artists and architects share your birth sign because while many of the more flamboyant signs are spouting out their ideas with enthusiasm, you are quietly turning dreams into reality, words into books and blueprints into buildings. You are also realistic enough to recognise the truth in the statement that a work of art tends to be nine tenths hard work and one tenth inspiration.

No matter what you try to do, you apply yourself with tremendous determination and are usually constructive and persevering, so may excel in more than one area. You dislike wasting time or being idle, so it is to be expected that you want to put your off-duty moments to good use. You will, therefore, consider the time you spend on body-care and exercise as worthwhile.

It is likely that you will become something of an authority on any subject that holds your interest. This thoroughness allows many Capricorns to earn extra income from a favourite hobby. Work first and play later is a Capricorn philosophy but too much work and not enough play can be bad for you. You must strive to maintain a fair balance between social and pleasurable pursuits, and work-related activities because you may be tempted to neglect the lighter side of life and the company of friends, due to becoming too absorbed in your latest project.

You are more of a mixer and a party-goer than some people realise, but prefer to stay in the background or on the fringe of the crowd unless you are called upon to entertain or take an active part. Parties and social gatherings can pose a serious threat to your weight loss intentions figure because of your genuine liking for good food. You are especially vulnerable to the risk of incorrect eating when faced with foods that were on your past list of favourites.

Your diet intentions can be threatened when you go on a holiday because this is one time you are ready to throw caution to the wind and seek adventure and new places to explore. Even if you intend to be very firm with yourself in the food department it is possible that you will come unstuck. This is because exotic places tend to have exotic menus, so special thought must be given to the fattening implications of the food you put on your plate.

AQUARIUS

20th JANUARY TO 18th FEBRUARY

Although Aquarius is not a particularly bright constellation, it is made up of a number of interesting stars.

Aquarius is the eleventh sign of the zodiac and symbolised by The Water Bearer, who carries a pitcher – representing Man carrying knowledge. Two planets co rule Aquarius. One is Uranus, the planet of sudden happenings, which is also associated with independence and revolution, and the other is Saturn, the planet of structure. Aquarius is the 'fixed' Air sign, suggesting that although Aquarians have an airy restlessness, they also seek stability. In common with the other Air signs of Gemini and Libra, Aquarians need the freedom to circulate and to communicate their thoughts and ideas. Considered to be the sign of Humanity, the Aquarian individual tends to possess a strong social conscience. Indeed it is by making a positive contribution to their community, that they find their true purpose.

YOUR SLIMMING PERSONALITY

There are so many contradictions in your nature that others may be forgiven if they find it hard to understand you. Even your two planetary rulers are diverse in nature, because Uranus is a planet connected with change, originality and freedom, while Saturn is associated with limitation, patience and learning life's lessons the hard way. This curious mixture of planetary strengths can now be used in your favour, because they are precisely the qualities you need to make a successful slimmer. Not only are you independent enough to refuse to stay, like a prisoner, bound to your fat, you are realistic enough to appreciate the sense of an organised diet-plan created with your personality in mind.

It's likely that you had a contrary streak in your nature from the time you were a child, because, as an Aquarian, you are a free spirit who resists doing what others want you to do, unless it coincides with what you want as well. No doubt, you are viewed by some as a person who makes their own rules and choices in life. You now have the sort of choice that is easy to make since it provides a real chance to break free from any bad eating patterns. You can look forward to liberating the inner you, the one who is slim and dynamic. From the moment you make your mind up to tackle your weight problem, you will be on the way to wearing a smaller size in clothes because once you reach a decision, you usually pursue it with energy and conviction.

YOUR SLIMMING STRENGTHS

You eat to live, rather than live to eat, which makes you an ideal candidate for a slimming diet. Here lies one of your greatest strengths in your fight against flab because it means that food doesn't dominate your thoughts and thereby constantly stimulate your

> ## HIT THAT HABIT
> Although you're interested in new ideas, you can sometimes be a slave to old habits when it comes to your choice of food. It would be a pity to eat the same selection of vegetables all through life. Your diet plan lasts for seven days so why not favour different vegetables on each one of them? Make a pact with yourself to experiment while slimming and look around for new shapes and flavours.

appetite. As a busy Aquarian, you have plenty of interests other than your stomach. There are always a multitude of things to do and people to see. You will also appreciate the merits of a diet plan that makes your life flow more smoothly, due to the knowledge that this new eating plan eliminates the hassle of wondering what to buy for the next meal. This applies even if you're one of the packed-lunch brigade, or if you need to snatch meals as and when possible, according to your schedule. You can now eat at home or away without the worry that your figure will suffer as a consequence.

You are honest with yourself, which is another great slimming strength. You are also prepared to accept the consequences of your own actions. Whenever your tape measure tells you that your current dimensions are "stretching" it a bit, or your weight is not to your liking or your doctor's, you are unlikely to blame it on depression or bad luck. This willingness to take responsibility for your life and what you eat is vital for any slimming regime to work, and it will save you from repeating any mistakes. Not only are you able to analyse the effects that others have on your eating patterns, you can also pin-point the types of situation that are bad for your figure.

Another plus factor, which will help tremendously in your efforts to lose weight, is the fact that you are your own person and not likely to be influenced by kindly, or come to that, scathing comments on how you look. The decision to take positive action about losing weight is one you will make for yourself. Once it is made, little will stand in your way.

If you're a true blue Aquarian, you also know your own worth and, at the same time, can quickly weigh up others. You rarely undersell yourself and whether you're negotiating money, love or chores, you know when not to compromise. This sense of self-worth can be the spur you need to stick rigidly to a sensible, new eating pattern, rather than indulging in quick but forbidden bites. Fortunately, you more than most are willing to wait for the results you seek, which means that the outer you stands every chance of becoming a true reflection of the inner you, which is slim, fit and full of the joys of life.

Aquarius is one of the three "fixed" signs, which signifies that there is a fixed, stubborn side to your nature. This is another strength because it gives you the tenacity to carry on dieting and exercising until you've reached the exact weight and size you have in mind. Although you need to be convinced that a new idea will work before you'll dive in at the deep end, once you committed yourself, you will give it your best shot, which is all you need to do now!

You are likely to hold strong views of what is right and wrong, and you are ready to fight for any cause you believe in, especially if it is a cause that helps people in general. The right that everyone has to be proud of their body and to feel good about themselves, is a cause to support at the moment, but you need to start with your own body, bearing in mind that example is the best teacher. Aquarius is considered to be one of the most fair-minded signs of the zodiac and "equality" is a key word in the Aquarian vocabulary. You may now wish to let it be known to your family and friends that you consider it as important for men, as it is for women, to keep fit and look good.

YOUR SLIMMING WEAKNESSES

One of your greatest slimming weaknesses is your tendency to "make do" with food that's instantly available. In your book eating means refuelling and is a necessity rather than a grand passion. This means you grab a quick sandwich or eat up yesterday's left-overs, whatever they may be, when hungry, because whatever's going will serve the purpose of filling you up. The next time you feel like tucking into the remains of last night's sweet and sour, or apple tart, remember that you could soon be wearing any excess calories consumed.

Instant food may temporarily satisfy your stomach,

SPONSORED SLIMS

Yours is the sign considered to be the most socially conscious of the zodiac, so why not organise a sponsored slim? While you're shedding weight, which you're better off without anyway, you will have the added pleasure of knowing you're raising money for the fight against hunger and poverty in other parts of the world.

FRUITY FEASTS

Some fruits go well with savoury foods. Try these tasty combinations as a starter or as your main course: orange with chicken, melon with cottage cheese, pineapple with ham or apple with tuna. Fruit for breakfast is also a very healthy way to start the day. Eat it on its own or chop a small quantity into a bowl of cereal for added fibre.

---

but it doesn't take long for your body's computer to do its sums and calculate whether its latest input contains sufficient nutrients and vitamins. If it doesn't, beware! Before you know it, that empty feeling will hit you again and your appetite and waistline will both grow larger and larger.

Avoid falling into another Aquarian classic slimming trap. This is one of rushing to the nearest food store to buy essentials, such as milk or bread, and staggering out laden down with an assortment of biscuits, crisps, nuts, pies and other instantly edible foods. It is advisable to stay well away from shops and supermarkets unless you are armed with a carefully prepared shopping list. This should be compiled after you've eaten a meal and before the next meal becomes imminent. Shopping impulsively will incline you to

---

SALAD CRAZE

Are your salads dreary? A few lettuce leaves and slices of cucumber, and a tomato? Then it's definitely time for a change! Mix a whole new range of tastes and try new dressings too, such as vinegar and lemon juice with fresh herbs. You could also use cold pasta as the basis for a main course salad, and serve with tuna or chopped chicken.

---

shop unwisely and buy food that is of the wrong type.

Yet another of your slimming obstacles, is that the Uranian energy that is so strong in your birth chart, stirs you up every now and again, and urges you to experiment and rebel against too many rules and regulations. Following a recipe closely is not really your style, so whether the results are mouth watering or delegated to the dog to eat, you can claim that every dish you concoct is an exclusive. Try to curb that adventurous streak a little and stay safely within the range of the suggested foods and portions. This is the only certain way to achieve your required weight loss, without a set-back. Your weight loss plan has been carefully calculated and balanced. Meanwhile, start planning the changes in your wardrobe in order to suit the reduced you that's on the way.

YOU AND YOUR BODY

There are probably so many thoughts buzzing around in your head at any given moment that you sometimes fail to hear the messages given by your inner workings, so make a point of trying to listen to what your body is telling you from one meal to the next. There's no point in fooling yourself that you can keep putting off until tomorrow the sensible eating that must be done today. Do you find yourself putting off vital health and dental appointments because you're too busy in other directions? A tendency to 'live in your head' can be a contributory cause to problems arising in your general well-being. It can also threaten your chances of becoming slim and fit.

You, more than most, need to cultivate good habits relating to your health. Dieting needs to become part

---

HEAD FOR HERBS

Where tea and coffee are concerned, there's no need to always be a milk and sugar merchant (both add extra calories to drinks). Instead, treat yourself to a selection of herbal teas. Jasmine and peppermint are particularly refreshing. If you hanker for familiar tastes, compromise with black coffee or tea with lemon and you will never look back.

---

of your way of life, so that your body is always stocked up with the essential vitamins and minerals that keep you charged with energy and glowing with health.

The circulation, and the ankles and calves are the parts of the body particularly associated with Aquarius. This implies that you should take special care of your legs and guard against such weight-related conditions as varicose veins. Skipping, jogging and aerobic exercises are representative of the sort of movements that can keep you in shape. Challenge your body with progressive exercise, rather than throwing yourself into a vigorous work out from day one and try to exercise daily. This can consist of a brisk ten-minute walk, a stint of gardening or some energetic housework, building up to longer periods. Daily exercise speeds up the metabolism, so surplus weight will drop away, as if by magic. The fact is that a once-a-week workout has little effect on your regular weight.

In keeping with those born under Gemini and Libra, the two other Air signs, you benefit from plenty of fresh air so, whatever the weather, don't forget to include plenty of outdoor activities in your programme.

YOU AND YOUR EMOTIONS

In affairs of the heart, you look for a friend first, a lover second, because friendship is everything to you. You hate to lose a single pal, so are the world's worst at closing the door on a broken romance. Your philosophy is that a relationship doesn't end, it merely changes. Luckily for you, your appetite is rarely influenced by the state of your love life and whether you are giddy with excitement about a brand new passion, comfortably "settled down" or still looking, you are able to munch food steadily through the sort of emotional dramas that knock other people's diet intentions for six. This is because you refuse to be a slave to your passions and only alter your eating patterns if and when it suits you to do so.

Many Aquarians marry young, usually before they become set in their ways. It can be hard for you to commit yourself again if your first attempts at finding wedded bliss fail. Subconsciously or not, you tend to search for an exact clone of your first love and it takes some Aquarians most of their lives to wake up to the fact that they will either have to remarry the same person or accept a different model. Ideally your partner must be slightly unpredictable. Sensible one minute but zany the next. They must also be intelligent without being a know-all because you can't stand pompous people. Above all, they must be self-sufficient because you shy away from anyone who is too clinging. This is because you dislike to be pinned down or too committed. Even so, a commitment is called for now if you are to achieve the size and weight you desire.

You respond positively to those born under the

other Air signs of Gemini, Libran as well as your fellow Aquarians. This mix often works extremely well in a long-term relationship because it is a marriage of the minds. Not only do you speak the same language, there will always be plenty to talk about. You know how to respond to each other and you also respect each other's right to space and freedom, which means you will be happy when socialising apart, as well as together. If you start slimming with someone born under an Air sign, expect to share lots of laughs, as well as a wealth of interesting thoughts and ideas.

One thing you share with a Taurus, Virgo or Capricorn, the Earth sign people, is the ability to be realistic about the potential of your association. If you have enough in common and decide to get together, you could go far together. An Earth sign partner will provide the back-up you need for your slimming regime, especially when you go through highly-pressurised periods. At the same time, you can draw them out of themselves and help them to break down the reserves that Earth sign people tend to have, which may deprive them of the fun and lighter side of life. You can also encourage your Earth companions to think positively about the joy of being slim.

Those born under Aries, Leos and Sagittarius, the three fire signs, are compatible with your own birth sign. Like you, they enjoy social inter-action and new challenges. In a romantic relationship, there will be plenty of sparkle at first, but you must be prepared to work at it if you hope to keep the love light burning brightly. Their enthusiasm to race ahead all the time could bring out the most stubborn side of your personality. Even so, you can count on the Fire sign members of your household to rally round when you announce your intentions of following a weight loss plan. Indeed, unless they are thin, expect them to want to join in and show you how it is done.

It is a curious fact, that although a relationship with a person born under a Water sign, i.e. a Cancer, Scorpio or Pisces, is never without its share of problems, you are irresistibly drawn to these signs and may therefore be married to, or have a Water sign person as one of your closest friends. Their uncanny intuition and sensitive feelings intrigue you, and their ability to sense the mood of the moment and know when you are upset or overwrought never fails to astonish you.

You will both love and hate the caring a Water-sign partner offers because your basic urge, which is to move unfettered by restriction, is threatened by a clinging Water-vine, who's natural instinct is to belong to and hang on tightly. Nevertheless, you could be pleasantly surprised if you enlist their help as a slimming supporter. You'll receive bags of encouragement, plus welcome assistance with shopping and meal preparation. You'll also be the recipient of well-meaning but unwanted advice and sympathy, which you will probably loathe!

If you decide to diet independently, watch out for sabotage because Water sign people resent feeling unneeded!

YOUR CREATIVE ENERGIES
There's nothing you like more than a brain-teaser because you get a kick out of being able to resolve a

CONSUMER NEWS
Be smart and arrange to eat with a fellow Aquarius, or Gemini or Libran when you lack stimulus in your day. You'll be so busy swapping news, stimulating good ideas and interesting information, that there will be scant time left for nibbling or contemplating the contents of the fridge.

problem. There's also a competitive edge to your personality, so you look for stimulus or even a degree of challenge in your leisure activities. Start your weight loss plan now and it won't be long before you can tell your friends and family that once again, you have taken positive action to overcome a weight problem.

Next time you pass the first-aid person, the school crossing officer or the assistant in the local charity shop, stop and take a second look. Do they seem familiar? It wouldn't be surprising if they did because the chances are they are fellow Aquarians. Many natives of your sign enjoy spending part of their leisure time in work that will help others, and it's likely that you have at least one spare-time activity that is useful to the community. This means that a sponsored slim is right up your street because nothing pleases you more than knowing that one of the spin offs of losing weight is being able to do some good for a favourite charity.

You enjoy the security of having a large circle of friends on which to call, because they can rescue you when you fall into one of your regular spells of deep loneliness, which although rarely lasting for long, represents one of the more stressful times for your figure. It is to your advantage to follow as many of your creative interests as possible in group situations, or with at least one companion.

Even so, and although Aquarius is one of the most group-conscious signs of the zodiac, social eating can pose a problem. You should be especially attentive to the impact the typical fare served up at a barbecue or garden party has on your waistline. Pack your diet meal into a picnic basket and you can stay figure-conscious whenever you find that you are eating out of doors.

You rarely allow sentiment to sway your judgement so your friends and associates tend to look your way when they want a straight answer to a question, knowing that they will receive unbiased and well-considered advice. It comes easy for you to supply the obvious answer if a heavy-weight friend is worried about their increasing girth, but you can be strangely resistant to taking advice yourself, unless you have asked for it specifically.

Projects that allow you to add a personal touch to them, such as model making, specialist cooking and astrology may hold special appeal. You also possess a practical slant, so may be adept at a number of different handicrafts. You are also fascinated by such things as astrology, as well as modern technology, and may well use computers and similar devices at both work and play. The freedom to explore and experiment is important to you.

Like the Water Bearer that symbolises your Air sign, you are attracted to water and may find boating, rowing, canoeing or sailing ideal ways to spend a vacation. You are willing to "rough it" a little in order to go somewhere unusual or unconventional; that is providing it allows you to be with other people. An off-beat, action-packed holiday is far more to your taste than being idle and it is also less likely to result in you nibbling away the time out of boredom.

Your bathroom and kitchen scales not to mention your can-opener, mobile phone and toothbrush, are probably an update on everyone else's. This is because out of all the twelve signs of the zodiac, yours is the most inventive and eager to try what is new or different. This bodes well for your weight loss campaign which is designed to suit your zodiac group.

PISCES

19th FEBRUARY TO 20th MARCH

Although Pisces is not a particularly bright constellation in the night sky, it is nevertheless, one of the easiest to identify because it looks like a 'V' in the night sky.

Pisces is the twelfth and last sign of the zodiac, and is symbolised by two fish, which are usually depicted tied together by a cord but swimming in opposite directions. This represents the duality that's at the heart of every Pisces. This dual theme is reinforced by the fact that there are two planetary rulers for Pisces. One is Jupiter, the largest of the planets, which is associated with expansion and opportunity. The other is Neptune, the planet of dreams, inspiration and ideals. Pisces is a mutable (adaptable) water sign and the Pisces individual is considered to be highly sensitive, imaginative and impressionable.

YOUR SLIMMING PERSONALITY

The two fish, which symbolise your sign, are usually depicted pulling away from each other; representing dual desires. When the time comes to examine your dreams and be honest about which have a chance of being realised and those that will never to be anything more than wishful thinking, and so need to be put behind you, it can cause much inner turmoil and conflict. If you reflect on the pattern of events in your life you will probably agree that you have often found yourself having to choose between two options. This has forced you to decide on whether to swim up or downstream, when you may have preferred to do both. The fact that you're reading this book indicates that you are well aware of the right choice to make this time around, which is to start your weight loss campaign.

Your appearance is matter of importance where you're concerned because you are very sensitive to the impression you make on others, so what are you waiting for? Take the plunge, knowing that your diet has been carefully planned for your zodiac sign group. In due course you will be congratulating yourself on having made this particular choice.

Crash dieting is definitely not for you. The diet plan given in this book suits your need for a balanced and easy to follow eating pattern. It will allow you to achieve your desired size without undue hardship.

Although you may be reluctant to admit to your friends, at least initially, that you're beginning a new diet regime (you do like to keep your little secrets) once you start to hear favourable comments on the way you are slimming down, it will act like a spur to your resolve.

YOUR SLIMMING STRENGTHS

Pisces people are sometimes accused of being wishy-washy or vague and indecisive but this is not really the case. You're far tougher and more stubborn than some people may think, so even if trying to lose

> **BE PREPARED**
> Have a grand sort-out of your wardrobe in readiness for your new, slimmer look. Make two separate piles, the clothes that will suit you later because they can be revamped or taken in, and those that are definitely designed for heavy-weights. Plan to take these to the charity shop or pass them on to a hard up, but tubby friend.

weight seems daunting at times, you already possess the inner strength and resolve to get there in the end.

Those born under your imaginative sign are reputed to be the dreamers of the zodiac. In childhood you may have lived in a world of fantasy and played endless games of make-believe. However, it is now within your power to turn one particular dream into a reality. This is a dream than many Pisces people possess, which is to be slim and graceful. It remains to be said that there is a lot of truth in the saying that you have to have a dream to make a dream come true.

Receiving approval means a great deal to any Pisces, so you will probably go to tremendous lengths to win the respect and approval of those you admire. This need to prove yourself to others is a positive slimming advantage. The anticipation of being able to look into the mirror and congratulate yourself on what you see, knowing that other people will like what they see as well, will encourage you to stay on your diet, even when temptation of the edible type is strong.

Pisces are the poets of the zodiac because they are blessed with a vivid imagination and a steady flow of inspired ideas. This is another asset for a slimmer. Start visualising the attractive and fashionable clothes you will be able to wear once you have reached your target weight. Positive thought and visualisation can be used to your advantage in many ways so at this point keep seeing yourself in total control of your eating patterns.

Pisces was considered by the ancient astrologers to be the sign of self-sacrifice, partly due to the observation that Pisces people often went without in order to give to others. This can be used as a slimming strength because you can give the boxes of chocolates and other fattening goodies in your larder to some of your slimmer friends. Some sacrifices are well worth making, which applies when it comes to trying to lose weight. Keep reminding yourself that it is to your own advantage to look after your body and make sure that it's in good shape.

YOUR SLIMMING WEAKNESSES

One of your slimming obstacles is a tendency to procrastinate. You sometimes put things off, not because you're lazy but because you're afraid of failure. Fear of failure as well as of the unknown has caused many Pisces to sentence themselves to a life of

---

FOOD FOR THE SOUL

Music is very therapeutic to you, so the next time you feel tempted to raid your refrigerator for a slice of quiche or a savoury snack, first try playing a selection of opera, classical or pop favourites. The chances are that this will take your mind off food and give you a feeling of being complete.

frustration and compromise, in the mistaken belief that "the devil they know" is better than taking a chance.

The wish to slim down may be one you have had for a long time. You may have even felt depressed about your size and shape. However, instead of doing something about it, you may have chosen to pretend to your friends and colleagues that you were happy with the state of play. In your heart of hearts, you know that action needs to be taken if you are to free yourself from unwanted weight.

The truth is that you are rarely motivated to make a change until you are confident that it will be for the best. However, the results that will be apparent even after only one short week will give you a taste of what is to come. Expect to enjoy a steady weight loss as well as a general boost in your energy levels and sense of well-being.

The gentle side of your nature means that you can find it hard to be firm with others, and by the same token, you can also find it hard to be firm with yourself. As you know, the sight of a mouth-watering slice of pie, or other delicacy, just begging to be eaten, is a real test of will power! Keep leftovers in containers that you can't see through and you will not be bombarded with visual temptations whenever you open the fridge. This will also help you to wait until it is time for your next meal.

As Pisces is one of the three Water signs, (the others are Cancer and Scorpio), water is your natural element. What you drink is as important to your weight as what you eat. If you are in the habit of sipping liquids between meals, give due consideration

SNACK ATTACK

The small snacks tend to be your downfall, so if you have been inclined to nibble your way through the day, stop now! Set times and select places where food is banned! Even better, indulge in activities of the sort that make eating impractical or anti-social.

to their calorific content. Take care because the wrong drinks can be secret enemies by expanding your waistline without filling your stomach. Quench your thirst with a cocktail of natural water and a splash of lemon, lime or orange, rather than drinking a double measure of a sugary soft drink that can jeopardise your best slimming efforts.

Yours is an especially sensitive sign and it's also likely that you are telepathic. You may often know who is on the other end of the 'phone before you have picked up the receiver, or what someone is going to say before they say it. You respond instinctively to others and possess a natural gift of being able to fathom out the mood of the moment and know what is really going on. Rather like a sponge, you soak up impressions and moods. This can be counter-productive to your weight loss efforts, because you could find yourself organising the meal that your partner or family is thinking about, whether or not it's bad news for your diet. Keep reviewing your actions to ensure that what you are eating has not been unduly influenced by the likes and dislikes of those you care about the most.

As you are particularly influenced by the moods and dictates of others, also make a point of surrounding yourself with positive, energetic people while you're slimming. On no account should you dine with anyone who tries to dominate you, especially with regards to what you should eat.

Also beware of those who think that they know what's good for you unless they possess expert knowledge. This particularly applies if they are overweight themselves, because they may fail to understand that the four square meals a day, that suits them, is not, or is no longer, your style.

YOU AND YOUR BODY

Jupiter, associated with growth and expansion, is one of the co-rulers of Pisces. Like those born under Sagittarius, the other sign ruled by this benevolent planet, you can find yourself expanding literally as you grow older, with your waistline expanding a little more each year of your life.

The parts of the body ruled by Pisces are the feet and toes, so pamper your feet and give them all the loving care they deserve. Swollen ankles, corns, bunions and blisters, not to mention tender or burning heels and soles, are all part of the overweight problem so well-fitting shoes are an essential part of your wardrobe. Pinched toes will soon make their

---

JUST IMAGINE
Use your vivid imagination to make every single meal a brand new experience. Sprinkle ginger or cinnamon on fruit, add black peppercorns to fish, a dash of chilli to meat, oregano on tomatoes or cheese and marjoram to pasta. Also ring the changes in the way you present your food, so that your meal is always of interest and pleasing to the eye!

TABLE FOR ONE

If you eat alone most of the time, make a habit of laying the table and sitting down for your meal. This is important because you will then feel as if you have had a proper meal. You could remain unsatisfied if you make do with a hurried snack and eat it standing or while you continue to be absorbed in other activities.

uncomfortable presence felt and that Pisces smile will fade if your feet are killing you, which is exactly what will happen if the weight stacked up on top of them keeps growing heavier and threatens to overload them! When you start to reduce your inches, don't be surprised if your toes curl up with pleasure, especially when you treat yourself to fashionable shoes that are designed for a slim person rather than a fat one.

Like it does for those born under Cancer and Scorpio, the other two Water signs, your weight tends to fluctuate according to what is going on in your life, so resist any temptation you may have to jump on to your bathroom scales every single day. You'll obtain a more accurate picture of your progress by weighing in once a week at a regular time. Bear in mind that it is the steady, constant effort invested in a weight loss campaign that brings appreciable and lasting results.

Many Pisces love to dance. Even if you're not an aspiring ballroom or disco champion, you will find that exercising to rhythm is good for you. It is a fun and effective way of shaping up and shedding that surplus weight. Neptune, one of your planetary rulers, rules music, so music is particularly important to a Pisces. It takes you out of yourself and helps you relax while you throw off the tensions of the day. Exercise routines that are enjoyable are a must for you because you can quickly lose heart if slimming means suffering.

Learning to live in the present is one of the Pisces challenges in life. Instead of reminiscing about how slim you were once, or speculating on how slim you might have been "if only", assess your body as it is today and decide how you want it to look, and start your diet and exercise plan now!

YOU AND YOUR EMOTIONS

Yours is a romantic sign and you love to be in love. **The good news is that flirting and falling in love works wonders for your figure!** The excitement, the sheer pleasure, the teasing, the chase and being close to someone special makes any thoughts of over-eating fly out of the window.

However, some Pisces spend their entire lifetime pining for the love that they have lost or dreaming about the love that they long for but which may never be. If you give your heart, you give it completely and often paint a glowing picture in your mind's eye of the one you have chosen, refusing to see their failings. When your emotions are involved, you tend to wear rose tinted spectacles and can therefore, become disillusioned with the passage of time. If this should happen, you can become too exacting and too critical of anyone else who comes along. Guard against any inclination to turn to food and drink for comfort if the person you devoted yourself has let you down.

You offer sympathy and caring and are ready to

make sacrifices for those who matter to you, such as your spouse or family. Ideally, you need a mate who is protective and supportive, as well as understanding and practical enough to lend a hand in times of crisis.

If someone in your family or circle of friends is born under one of the three Fire signs of Aries, Leo or Sagittarius, you will have realised that they tackle life in a very different way to you. They take the bold, direct approach and can be very assertive, while your way is subtle and gently persuasive.

When it comes to joining up with a Fire sign person in your weight loss campaign, you could just succeed where they fail. This is because impatience is a common failing in the Fire sign personalities, who seek instant results. This is not the way it works because fat cells burn less energy than muscles, so the way to reduce is by establishing new and healthy, long-term eating habits.

Those born under one of the three Air signs of Gemini, Libra and Aquarius, may represent a challenge to you, but not as much of a challenge as you do to them. Your ultra-sensitivity, which makes you easily hurt, and your ability to be evasive so that no one knows what you're planning, will bother and bewilder curious Air signs.

These people prefer to rationalise their thoughts, feelings and actions, so may be surprised with the way that you can, without asking a single question, make accurate assessments. Together, you would make a restless combination. You would achieve most if you both work towards a common aim. Unless this is the case, a Pisces and an Air-sign person are likely to become absorbed in the sort of interests that cause them to drift apart, without fully appreciating the depths in each other.

A partner born under one of the three Earth signs of Taurus, Virgo or Capricorn, will provide stability and solid support. They will help you to identify and realise your main aims in life. You are naturally sympathetic to each other, so this relationship could work well and prove beneficial when it come to losing weight. You will soon sense it if your Earth partner or friend is in danger of breaking their diet, so will be able to use your powers of persuasion to keep them on track. They are likely to reorganise your larder, refrigerator or freezer, so you will know exactly what's in stock, what to throw out and what to add to your shopping list.

Living with one of the Water sign people, which are Pisces, Cancer or Scorpio, should prove mutually beneficial. You offer comfort and emotional support for each other and there is likely to be a quiet, relaxed empathy between you. This provides a sound basis for a long-term partnership. The biggest problem you may have to contend with is your sensitivity to each other's moods. If one of you is not on top form, it can affect the other one and pose a mutual threat to your diet intentions.

WINNING WATER
Pisces is a water sign and water is a winner for you when it comes to choosing a drink. Sipping water can curb the appetite and satisfy the need to have 'something' in between meals. Serve the water in an attractive glass and add a slice of lemon or lime because this will turn even plain old tap water into a classy tipple.

YOUR CREATIVE ENERGIES

Many Pisces are blessed with great inspiration, which adds a special quality to their work, so it follows that Pisces men and women swell the ranks of the artists, poets, actors and musicians of society. Apart from obvious artistic pursuits, there are many other ways in which you are likely to express your creative energies, for instance through gardening, decorating, handicrafts and various forms of D.I.Y. The urge to create is very strong in you, and it is by developing this creative side of your personality that you gain a sense of inner peace and tranquillity, and find fulfilment.

That ability you have to lose yourself in whatever is on your mind is another reason to make your creative activities important. You are less likely to nibble when busy creating a work of art, but you might be tempted to do so while watching someone else creating a masterpiece on the television.

You need plenty of music in your life because listening to music, playing it, or singing or dancing along with it, uplifts your spirits and puts you in a good frame of mind. This is particular the case if you are one of those gifted Pisces who composes music or plays a musical instrument, such as a keyboard, violin or guitar.

Your artistic efforts, whether used for work or play, allow you to express your intense inner feelings in a positive and enjoyable way. Overeating and other excesses, such as excessive smoking or drinking alcohol, are usually a form of escapism. Your key to maintaining a constant weight and a healthy body is to create a happy and interesting life for yourself.

Although you, more than most, need periods on your

own, so that you can repair the damage done to your nerves by the frantic pace of the world, guard against becoming too much of a loner or stop-at-home.

It's especially beneficial for you to participate in group activities at times. A keep-fit class would be especially good or, as befits your natural sense of rhythm, a dancing class. You often do well in sports and activities that depend on good balance such as skiing, skating, yoga and certain water sports.

You cannot cope with discord or too much hassle, so you need to plan your off-duty moments carefully, especially your holidays. Opt for places that offer peace, tranquillity and beauty when arranging a vacation or mini-break. Uncomfortable accommodation or ugly surroundings is something to avoid at all costs. If you feel uncertain of where to go, trust your intuition to guide you because it rarely lets you down.

THE
ASTRODIETS

THE DIET FOR FIRE SIGNS
(ARIES, LEO, SAGITTARIUS)

This diet allows you six meals a day, and yet will result in a speedy weight loss. Surprisingly, perhaps, eating more often can be a very effective way to slim – because it keeps your metabolism "revved up" and stops your system from feeling and reacting as if it were being starved of supplies. Not only are the results quick – the meals on the diet are also quick and easy to prepare.

Once the week is up, you should return to normal eating, but of course you will have to watch your intake if your weight is not to shoot up again. So don't go back to bad old habits – use what you learn on this diet as a guide to healthy eating for the future.

On occasion, you can repeat any two days of the diet to offset a heavier-eating event – like Christmas- and help to keep your weight where you want it to be. However,do not repeat the diet in its entirety more frequently than once in every six weeks.

YOU MUST DRINK 6–8 GLASSES OF WATER EVERY DAY!

NOTE: It is always wise to check with your GP before starting on any diet particularly if you have a health problem.

DAY ONE

MEAL 1:

> 1 Weetabix with 1 banana, sliced and
> 4 fl. oz./125ml semi-skimmed milk; tea or
> coffee, black or with semi-skimmed milk,
> NO SUGAR (you may use a sweetener).

MEAL 2:

> 3 oz./75g grapes

MEAL 3:

> 4 oz./100g smoked mackerel, 1 tomato,
> 5oz. /125g.pot of diet coleslaw, 1 slice
> wholemeal bread.

MEAL 4:

> 8 oz./250g any combination of raw salad
> vegetables (choose from beetroot, cabbage,
> cauliflower, celery, chicory, cucumber,
> peppers, radishes, spring onions).

MEAL 5:

> 2 low-fat sausages, grilled and served
> with 4 oz./100g canned chopped tomatoes
> and 2 oz./50g brown rice, boiled.

MEAL 6:

> 1 apple
> In addition: 2 cups tea or coffee, black or
> with semi-skimmed milk, NO SUGAR
> (you may use a sweetener).

DAY TWO

MEAL 1:

1 oz./25g bran cereal with 1/2oz./12g
sultanas and 4 fl. oz./125 ml semi-
skimmed milk; tea or coffee, black
or with semi-skimmed milk, NO SUGAR
(you may use a sweetener).

MEAL 2:

2 satsumas

MEAL 3:

2-slice wholemeal sandwich of
1 teaspoon low-fat spread mixed with
2 oz./50g Edam cheese, grated, and 1
tablespoon tomato ketchup plus
cucumber slices.

MEAL 4:

As Day One

MEAL 5:

2 low-fat beefburgers, grilled with
1 tomato, halved and grilled and
5 oz./125g baked beans in tomato sauce.

MEAL 6:

1 pear
In addition: 2 cups tea or coffee, black or
with semi-skimmed milk, NO SUGAR
(you may use a sweetener).

DAY THREE

MEAL 1:

1 Weetabix with 1 apple, chopped, and
4 fl. oz./125ml semi-skimmed milk;
tea or coffee, black or with semi-skimmed
milk, no SUGAR (you may use a sweetener).

MEAL 2:

2 oz./50g cottage cheese and 2 crispbreads

MEAL 3:

3 1/2 oz./90g tuna, canned in brine, with
2 oz./50g sweetcorn, drained, 4 oz./l00g
cold, cooked green beans, 2 oz./50g
canned red kidney beans, and 2 tables-
poons/30ml low-calorie vinaigrette
dressing.

MEAL 4:

As Day One

MEAL 5:

4 oz./l00g roast or baked chicken, NO
SKIN,with a 4 oz./l00g jacket-baked
potato, dressed with 1 tablespoon/15ml
low-fat natural yoghurt plus.4 oz./l00g
any green vegetable, steamed.

MEAL 6:

2 satsumas.
In addition: 2 cups tea or coffee, black or
with semi-skimmed milk, NO SUGAR
(you may use a sweetener).

DAY FOUR

MEAL 1:

1 oz./25g bran cereal with half oz./12g dried apricots, chopped, and 4 fl. oz./125ml semi-skimmed milk; tea or coffee, black or with semi-skimmed milk, NO SUGAR (you may use a sweetener).

MEAL 2:

3 oz./75g grapes

MEAL 3:

2-slice wholemeal sandwich of 1 hard-boiled egg, chopped and mixed with a punnet of mustard and cress and 1 tablespoon low-calorie salad cream.

MEAL 4:

As Day One

MEAL 5:

6 oz./150g white fish, grilled and served with lemon and parsley, plus 4 oz./l00g potatoes, boiled and 2 oz./50g peas, boiled.

MEAL 6:

3 slices of pineapple, fresh or tinned without sugar. In addition: 2 cups tea or coffee, black or with semi-skimmed milk, NO SUGAR (you may use a sweetener).

DAY FIVE

MEAL 1:

1 Weetabix with 1 banana, sliced and 4 fl. oz./125ml semi-skimmed milk; tea or coffee, black or with semi-skimmed milk, NO SUGAR (you may use a sweetener).

MEAL 2:

2 crispbreads spread with 1 teaspoon of Marmite and topped with 1 tomato, halved.

MEAL 3:

2-slice wholemeal sandwich of 1 slice lean ham with 1 processed cheese slice and lettuce.

MEAL 4:

As Day One

MEAL 5:

5 oz./125g jacket-baked potato, topped with 2 oz./50g cottage cheese and chives.

MEAL 6:

1 apple
In addition: 2 cups tea or coffee, black or with semi-skimmed milk, NO SUGAR (you may use a sweetener).

DAY SIX

MEAL 1:

1 egg, poached or boiled, and 1 slice
wholemeal bread or toast with a scraping
of low-fat spread; tea or coffee, black or
with semi-skimmed milk, NO SUGAR
(you may use a sweetener).

MEAL 2:

1 banana with 1 oz./25g chopped dates

MEAL 3:

1 oz./25g cold cooked pasta with
2 oz./50g cottage cheese and 4 black
olives, chopped in.

MEAL 4:

As Day One

MEAL 5:

4 1 oz./25g slices lean ham wrapped
around 4 sticks of pre-cooked broccoli
topped with 2 processed cheese slices and
browned under a hot grill, served with 2
oz./50g sweetcorn.

MEAL 6:

3 slices of pineapple, fresh or tinned
without sugar.
In addition: 2 cups tea or coffee, black or
with semi-skimmed milk, NO SUGAR
(you may use a sweetener).

DAY SEVEN

MEAL 1:

1 rasher lean bacon, grilled with 1
tomato, halved and grilled and 1 slice
wholemeal toast; tea or coffee, black or
with semi-skimmed milk, NO SUGAR
(you may use a sweetener).

MEAL 2:

1 slice of wholemeal bread or toast
spread with 1 teaspoon/5ml honey.

MEAL 3:

2 oz./50g prawns, mixed with 2 sticks
celery, chopped, and half a small apple,
chopped, and dressed with 1 teaspoon/
5ml low-calorie salad dressing and
1 teaspoon/ 5ml tomato ketchup plus
a dash of lemon juice, 1 slice wholemeal
bread.

MEAL 4:

As Day One

MEAL 5:

4 oz./100g liver, shredded and dry-fried
with half a small onion, chopped,
2 oz./50g mushrooms, sliced, and
1 tomato, skinned and chopped, served
with 2 oz./50g brown rice, boiled, and
4 oz./100g spinach, steamed.

MEAL 6:

Remaining half apple, chopped and served
with 1 small orange, segmented, 1 small
banana, sliced and 2 oz./ 50g grapes
sprinkled with a little fresh orange juice
In addition: 2 cups tea or coffee, black or
with semi-skimmed milk, NO SUGAR
(you may use a sweetener).

NOTE: You must eat the full quantity of salad
vegetables each day. However, if you find it too
much at a sitting, you may instead add a little to
other meal menus, or even snack on salad as
additional mini-meals.

THE DIET FOR EARTH SIGNS
(TAURUS, VIRGO, CAPRICORN)

This diet consists of three planned meals a day plus a treat. The diet, which is fairly strict, must be followed exactly apart from the optional daily treat which can be exchanged for some fresh fruit if you prefer. You can follow this diet for one to two weeks at a time and repeat as often as two weeks in every six. You must, of course, eat sensibly for the rest of the time. It's also essential to weigh and measure portions carefully and avoid resorting to guess-work.

YOU MUST DRINK 6-8 GLASSES OF WATER EVERY DAY!

NOTE: It is always wise to check with your GP before starting any diet – particularly if you have a health problem.

EVERY DAY you're allowed half a pint/300 ml of skimmed milk - in addition to any milk listed on the diet - and unlimited tea or coffee, using milk from the allowance, but NO SUGAR (you may use a sweetener) and 1 slice of wholemeal bread, in addition to any bread listed. Where no quantity is given for a vegetable, you may eat an unlimited amount.

DAY ONE

BREAKFAST:
>Half a grapefruit
>1 1/2oz./37g unsweetened bran or
>oat cereal
>4 fl. oz./125ml skimmed milk

LIGHT MEAL:
>2 oz./50g Edam cheese
>Salad vegetables
>1 granary roll
>1 apple

MAIN MEAL:
>31/2oz./90g bacon steak, grilled with
>1 pineapple ring and
>half a tomato

YOUR TREAT:
>1 doughnut

DAY TWO

BREAKFAST:

> 4 fl. oz./125 ml unsweetened orange juice
> 1 egg, poached,
> on 1 slice wholemeal toast with a
> scraping of low-fat spread

LIGHT MEAL:

> 2 oz./50g beefburger, grilled
> Salad vegetables
> 1 pear

MAIN MEAL:

> 6 oz./175g cod fillet, grilled with a
> scraping of low-fat spread
> 5 oz./125g potato, steamed or boiled
> French beans
> Carrots
> 1 low-fat fruit yoghurt

YOUR TREAT:

> 1 packet low fat crisps

DAY 3

BREAKFAST:
>4 fl. oz./125ml tomato juice
>1 rasher lean back bacon, grilled
>2 oz./50g mushrooms, simmered in stock
>1 slice wholemeal toast

LIGHT MEAL:
>31/2oz./90g can tuna in brine
>Salad vegetables
>1 orange

MAIN MEAL:
>4 oz./l00g liver, grilled
>11/2 oz./37g brown rice, boiled or steamed
>spinach
>Carrots
>8 oz./250g wedge of melon

YOUR TREAT:
>2 oz./50g chocolate

DAY FOUR

BREAKFAST:

Half a grapefruit
11/2 oz./37g unsweetened bran or
oat cereal
4 fl. oz./125ml skimmed milk

LIGHT MEAL:

2 oz./50g lean ham
Salad vegetables
3 oz./75g grapes

MAIN MEAL:

5 oz./150g chicken joint, baked, NO SKIN
4 oz./l00g jacket-baked potato, served
with 1 tablespoon/15ml low-fat natural
yoghurt
Cauliflower
Sweetcorn
Strawberries, in natural juice

YOUR TREAT:

1 currant bun or scone with a scraping of
low-fat spread

DAY FIVE

BREAKFAST:

> 4 fl. oz./125ml unsweetened orange juice
> 1 egg, boiled
> 1 slice wholemeal toast
> Scraping of low-fat spread

LIGHT MEAL:

> 4 oz./l00g baked beans in tomato sauce on
> 1 slice wholemeal toast
> 1 orange

MAIN MEAL:

> 6 oz./175g plaice, grilled with a
> scraping of low-fat spread
> 4 oz./l00g potato, steamed or boiled
> celery hearts
> Carrots
> Pineapple slices, in natural juice

YOUR TREAT:

> 2 oz./50g sweets

DAY SIX

BREAKFAST:

> 2 fishcakes, grilled
> 2 tomatoes, grilled

LIGHT MEAL:

> 4 oz./l00g cottage cheese
> Salad vegetables
> 1 apple

MAIN MEAL:

> 2 small lamb cutlets (maximum raw
> weight 4 oz./100g each),
> Grilled cauliflower
> Peas
> Carrots
> 8 oz./250g wedge of melon

YOUR TREAT:

> 2 oz./50g salted peanuts

DAY SEVEN

BREAKFAST:

2 eggs, scrambled with
1 tablespoon/15ml skimmed milk, and
scraping of low-fat spread

LIGHT MEAL:

Salad vegetables ONLY

MAIN MEAL:

4 oz./l00g lean roast beef in gravy
4 oz./l00g roast potatoes – cut in large
pieces
Brussels sprouts
Parsnips
2 oz./50g vanilla ice cream
1 peach, fresh or tinned without sugar

YOUR TREAT:

2oz./50g peppermint creams

THE DIET FOR AIR SIGNS
(GEMINI, LIBRA, AQUARIUS)

This is a do-it-yourself diet, so you may devise your own meals and snacks from the foods listed for each day – which have been balanced nutritionally and calorie counted, to ensure a healthy and effective weight loss. You may combine the foods in any way you wish, but you must only cook them as directed. For flavour, you may add seasonings, herbs or spices, clear stock, vinegar or lemon juice; and up to 1 tablespoon/15ml of low-calorie salad dressing, tomato ketchup or brown sauce each day. You are also allowed one sweet or alcoholic treat daily.
This is listed last, but you may have it at any time you wish.

Apart from these additions, do not eat anything other than the foods and beverages listed for each day – and do not omit any! (If there is an item which you are unable to tolerate, replace it with something from the same food group – i.e. replace protein with protein, carbohydrate with carbohydrate, etc – and of a similar calorie value.)

YOU MUST DRINK 6-8 GLASSES OF WATER EVERY DAY!

NOTE: lt is always wise to check with your GP before starting any diet particularly if you have a health problem.

DAY ONE

2-4 cups of tea, with lemon or semi-skimmed milk,
NO SUGAR (you may use a sweetener)
2-4 cups of coffee, black or with semi-skimmed milk,
NO SUGAR (you may use a sweetener)
4 fl. oz./125 ml unsweetened orange or
grapefruit juice
2 oz./50g unsweetened bran cereal
4 fl. oz./125 ml semi-skimmed milk
2 slices wholemeal bread or toast
1/2oz./12g low-fat spread
2 eggs (poached, boiled or cooked with low-fat
spread - allowance above)
Unlimited salad vegetables (choose from lettuce,
cucumber, celery, peppers, tomatoes, beetroot,
watercress, mustard and cress)
4 oz./l00g chicken, NO SKIN
(cooked any way except fried)
6 oz./150g potato, preferably with skin (steamed,
baked or boiled)
6 oz./150g any green vegetables (steamed)
4 oz./l00g carrots (steamed)
1 small pot low-fat natural yoghurt
1 pear
1 orange

TREAT:
1 4 fl. oz./125ml glass of any white wine

DAY TWO

2-4 cups of tea, with lemon or semi-skimmed milk,
NO SUGAR (you may use a sweetener)
2-4 cups of coffee, black or with semi-skimmed milk,
NO SUGAR (you may use a sweetener)
1 whole grapefruit
2 oz./50g muesli
4 fl. oz./125 ml semi-skimmed milk
2 slices wholemeal bread or toast
1/2oz./12g low-fat spread
4 oz./l00g cottage cheese
Unlimited salad vegetables (detailed on Day One)
6 oz./150g white fish (steamed, poached or baked)
6 oz./150g potato, preferably with skin (steamed,
baked or boiled)
6 oz./150g any green vegetables (steamed)
2 oz./50g canned sweetcorn
Half a melon
2-3 figs

TREAT:
1 Quaker Harvest Crunch or Harvest Chewy Bar,
any flavour

DAY THREE

2-4 cups of tea, with lemon or semi-skimmed milk,
NO SUGAR (you may use a sweetener)
2-4 cups of coffee, black or with semi-skimmed milk,
NO SUGAR (you may use a sweetener)
1 whole orange
2 oz./50g unsweetened bran cereal
4 fl. oz./125ml semi-skimmed milk
2 slices wholemeal bread or toast
1/2oz./12g low-fat spread
4oz./100g tuna canned in brine
Unlimited salad vegetables (detailed on Day One)
2oz./50g rice, preferably brown (boiled or steamed)
4oz./100g liver or kidneys
6 oz./150g any green vegetables (steamed)
3 oz./75g carrots (steamed)
2 oz./50g vanilla ice cream
4 oz./l00g raspberries, fresh, frozen or canned
(without sugar)
1 pear

TREAT:
1 pub measure (50ml/1/3gill) Cinzano, Dubonnet
or Martini

DAY FOUR

2-4 cups of tea, with lemon or semi-skimmed milk,
NO SUGAR (you may use a sweetener)
2-4 cups of coffee, black or with semi-skimmed milk,
NO SUGAR (you may use a sweetener)
4 fl. oz./125ml unsweetened orange or
grapefruit juice
2 slices wholemeal bread or toast
1/2oz./12g low-fat spread
2 tablespoons/30ml honey
Unlimited salad vegetables (detailed on Day One)
2 oz./50g pasta, preferably wholemeal
2 oz./50g Edam cheese
6 oz./150g tomatoes, fresh or canned
3 oz./75g lean ham
6 oz./150g any green vegetables (steamed)
1 apple
1 orange
1 oz./25g raisins

TREAT:
1 fun size Mars Bar or Milky Way

DAY FIVE

2-4 cups of tea, with lemon or semi-skimmed milk,
NO SUGAR (you may use a sweetener)
2-4 cups of coffee, black or with semi-skimmed milk,
NO SUGAR (you may use a sweetener)
1 whole grapefruit
2 oz./50g unsweetened bran cereal
4 fl. oz./125g semi-skimmed milk
2 slices wholemeal bread or toast
1/2 oz./12g low-fat spread
4 oz./100g cottage cheese
Unlimited salad vegetables (detailed on Day One)
2 oz./50g lean minced beef
2 oz./50g rice, preferably brown (steamed or boiled)
4 oz./100g any green vegetables, steamed
2 oz./50g red kidney beans, canned
4 oz./100g tomatoes, fresh or canned
4 oz./100g onion (boiled or baked)
1 small pot low-fat fruit yoghurt
1 banana
1/2 melon

TREAT:
1 4 fl. oz./125ml glass any red wine

DAY SIX

2-4 cups of tea, with lemon or semi-skimmed milk,
NO SUGAR (you may use a sweetener)
2-4 cups of coffee, black or with semi-skimmed milk,
NO SUGAR (you may use a sweetener)
1 whole orange
2 oz./50g muesli
4 fl. oz./125ml semi-skimmed milk
2 slices wholemeal bread or toast
1/2oz./12g low-fat spread
4 oz./l00g prawns
Unlimited salad vegetables (detailed on Day One)
4 oz./l00g chicken, NO SKIN (cooked any way except
fried)
6 oz./150g potato, preferably with skin (steamed,
baked or boiled)
6 oz./150g any green vegetables (steamed)
4 oz./l00g swede, turnip or parsnip (steamed)
4 oz./l00g grapes
1 peach, fresh or 6 oz./150g tinned without sugar

TREAT:
Pub measure (25ml/1/3gill) any liqueur

DAY SEVEN

2-4 cups of tea, with lemon or semi-skimmed milk,
NO SUGAR (you may use a sweetener)
2-4 cups of coffee, black or with semi-skimmed milk,
NO SUGAR (you may use a sweetener)
4 fl. oz./125ml unsweetened orange or grapefruit
juice
2 eggs (poached, boiled or cooked with low-fat
spread - allowance below)
1 slice wholemeal bread or toast
1/2oz./12g low-fat spread
Unlimited salad vegetables (detailed on Day One)
4 oz./l00g tuna, canned in brine
4 oz./l00g lean roast pork or beef, NO FAT
4 oz./l00g potato, preferably with skin (steamed,
baked or boiled) 6 oz./150g any green vegetables
(steamed)
6 oz./150g any root vegetables (steamed)
2 tablespoons/30ml fat-free gravy
1 apple
1 pear
1 orange.

TREAT:
1 Mr. Kipling French Fancy individual iced cake

THE DIET FOR WATER SIGNS
(CANCER, SCORPIO, PISCES)

This is a pick-and-choose diet.

Seven breakfasts, seven light meals and seven main meals are listed - and you can choose which you have and when you have them. And, in case there's a meal you don't like, you have choice.

You can change any one light or main meal and substitute it with another. You may also repeat the same breakfast every day if you wish, unless it is a breakfast of an egg, which can be repeated only twice at the most in one week; but otherwise you may stick to just one or two favourite breakfasts if you prefer.

Five of the light meals are suitable to pack and carry, if you work away from home, so you've no excuse not to follow the diet.

To stay slim after your dieting week, you can repeat any of the meal combinations on up to 4 days a week, and eat normally – not over the top – on the other days.

YOU MUST DRINK 6-8 GLASSES OF WATER EVERY DAY.

NOTE: It is always wise to check with your GP before starting any diet – and this is a must if you have a health problem.

BREAKFASTS

Half grapefruit
1 egg, boiled
3 crispbreads oz./12g low-fat spread
Tea or coffee, black or with semi-skimmed milk,
NO SUGAR (you may use a sweetener)

4 fl. oz./125ml unsweetened orange juice
2 oz./50g any cereal, unsweetened
4 fl. oz./125ml semi-skimmed milk
Tea or coffee, black or with semi-skimmed milk,
NO SUGAR (you may use a sweetener)

5 fl. oz./150ml tomato juice
5 oz/125g baked beans in tomato sauce on
1 slice wholemeal toast
Tea or coffee, black or with semi-skimmed milk,
NO SUGAR (you may use a sweetener)

4 fl. oz./125ml unsweetened grapefruit juice
2 fishcakes, grilled
1 tomato, grilled
Tea or coffee, black or with semi-skimmed milk,
NO SUGAR (you may use a sweetener)

Half a grapefruit
2 rashers lean bacon, grilled
2 oz./50g mushrooms, poached in water with a dash
of Worcester sauce
Tea or coffee, black or with semi-skimmed milk,
NO SUGAR (you may use a sweetener)

Half a grapefruit
2 slices wholemeal bread or toast
1/2 oz./12g low-fat spread
2 teaspoons/10ml jam, marmalade or honey
Tea or coffee, black or with semi-skimmed milk,
NO SUGAR (you may use a sweetener)

1 whole orange
1 slice wholemeal bread, spread with
1 teaspoon/5ml Marmite, and topped with
2 tomatoes, halved
Tea or coffee, black or with semi-skimmed milk,
NO SUGAR (you may use a sweetener)

LIGHT MEALS

4 oz./lOOg cottage cheese OR 2 oz./50g Edam cheese
Mixed salad vegetables of your choice
1 teaspoon/5 ml low-calorie salad dressing
1 slice wholemeal bread
Scraping of low-fat spread
1 piece any fresh fruit up to 5 oz./125g weight

2 oz./5Og prawns, dressed with 1 teaspoon/5ml
low-calorie salad dressing PLUS 1 teaspoon/5ml
tomato ketchup
Mixed salad vegetables of your choice
1 slice wholemeal bread
Scraping of low-fat spread
1 piece any fresh fruit up to 5 oz./125ml in weight

2 oz./50g lean ham
2 oz./50g cottage cheese
2 tomatoes
1 slice wholemeal bread
Scraping of low-fat spread
1 piece any fresh fruit up to 5 oz./125g in weight

31/2oz./90g tuna canned in brine
2 oz./5Og chopped celery
1 oz./25g chopped onion
Lettuce
1 teaspoon low-calorie salad dressing
1 slice wholemeal bread

Scraping of low-fat spread
1 piece any fresh fruit up to 5 oz./125g in weight

1 egg, hard-boiled
Half a punnet mustard and cress
1 teaspoon/5ml low-fat salad dressing
Lettuce
1 slice wholemeal bread
Scraping of low-fat spread
1 piece any fresh fruit up to 5 oz./125g in weight

4 fish fingers, grilled
2 oz./50g peas, boiled
1 tomato, halved and grilled
Mixed salad of any three fresh fruits, maximum
weight 8 oz./250g
2 oz./50g low-fat beefburger, fresh or frozen, grilled
5 oz./125g baked beans in tomato sauce
1 tomato, halved and grilled
Mixed salad of any three fresh fruits, maximum
weight 8 oz./250g

MAIN MEALS

3 1/2oz./90g gammon steak, topped with
1 slice pineapple, fresh or canned without sugar
1/2 tomato
1 1/2oz./37g brown rice, boiled with
half a small onion, chopped
half a tomato, skinned and chopped, and
1 oz./25g mushrooms, chopped
1 oz./25g sweetcorn
6 oz./l50g cabbage, shredded and steamed with
1/4 green pepper, de-seeded and sliced in strips
2 oz./50g vanilla ice cream

3 oz./75g cold,cooked lean pork, cubed
1 1/2oz./37g dried apricots, chopped (soaked
overnight in orange juice)
1 1/2oz/37g brown rice, boiled with
half a small onion, chopped
combined, and served on a bed of
6 oz./l50g spinach, steamed and shredded
1 low-fat fruit-flavoured yoghurt

6 oz./l50g breast of chicken, NO SKIN,baked in foil
spread with scraping of low-fat spread, with
1 teaspoon/5ml lemon juice
1 crushed clove of garlic, and
1 tablespoon/l5ml fresh parsley, chopped finely
4 oz./l00g broccoli, steamed
2 oz./50g carrots, steamed
5 oz./125g jacket-baked potato, served with

1 tablespoon/15 ml low-fat natural yoghurt
2 oz./50g vanilla ice cream
1 bag frozen cod in butter or parsley sauce
5 oz./125g jacket-baked potato
6 oz./l50g sliced green beans, steamed
3 oz./75g swede, diced and steamed
1 low-fat fruit-flavoured yoghurt
2 oz./50g lean minced beef, dry-fried with
4 oz./l00g canned chopped tomatoes with herbs
half a small onion, chopped, and served on
11/2oz./37g wholemeal spaghetti, boiled
2 oz./50g peas, boiled
2 oz./50g vanilla ice cream

6 oz./l50g any white fish, steamed or baked with
herbs.
4 oz./l00g potatoes, steamed
4 oz./l00g sliced green beans, steamed
4 oz./l00g carrots, steamed
2 oz./50g vanilla ice cream

4 oz./l00g lean braising beef, cooked with water to
cover,
1 teaspoon/5ml tomato puree and 1 bay leaf
4 oz./l00g carrots, sliced
4 oz./l00g potatoes, cut into chunks, and
1 small onion, sliced
6 oz./l50g leeks, steamed
1 low-fat fruit-flavoured yoghurt

THE
SUN SIGN
PERIODS

DO YOU KNOW YOUR SUN SIGN?

The sign of the zodiac under which you were born never changes. It is your Sun sign throughout your life. However, the Sun doesn't enter or leave the signs of the zodiac on the same day or at the same time each year. This is why the dates used in star columns are approximate.

If you were born on the cusp, i.e. around the day when the Sun changed signs, you should check your true sign in the following tables. First look up the year and month in which you were born. The zodiac sign shown in the second column is the sign that the Sun entered when it made its monthly change of signs. The time given is G.M.T so allow for summer time changes.

For example if you were born on 20th March 1932 before 19h 54m GMT you are a Pisces. If you were born after 19h 54m you are an Aries.

In the Month of	The Sun entered	1930		1931		1932		1933	
		Day	Hr min	Day	Hr min	Day	Hr min	Day	Hr min
January	Aquarius	20	18 33	21	00 18	21	06 07	20	11 53
February	Pisces	19	09 00	19	14 40	19	20 28	19	02 16
March	Aries	21	08 30	21	14 06	20	19 54	21	01 43
April	Taurus	20	20 06	21	01 40	20	07 28	20	13 18
May	Gemini	21	19 42	22	01 15	21	07 06	21	12 57
June	Cancer	22	03 53	22	09 28	21	15 23	21	21 12
July	Leo	23	14 42	23	20 21	23	02 18	23	08 05
August	Virgo	23	21 26	24	03 10	23	09 06	23	14 52
September	Libra	23	18 36	24	00 23	23	06 16	23	12 01
October	Scorpio	24	03 26	24	09 16	23	15 04	23	20 48
November	Sagittarius	23	00 35	23	06 25	22	12 10	22	17 54
December	Capricorn	22	13 40	22	19 30	22	01 14	22	06 58

In the Month of	The Sun entered	1934 Day	Hr min	1935 Day	Hr min	1936 Day	Hr min	1937 Day	Hr min
January	Aquarius	20	17 37	20	23 28	21	05 12	20	11 01
February	Pisces	19	08 02	19	13 52	19	19 33	19	01 21
March	Aries	21	07 28	21	13 18	20	18 58	21	00 45
April	Taurus	20	19 00	21	00 50	20	06 31	20	12 19
May	Gemini	21	18 35	22	00 25	21	06 07	21	11 57
June	Cancer	22	02 48	22	08 38	21	14 22	21	20 12
July	Leo	23	13 42	23	19 33	23	01 18	23	07 07
August	Virgo	23	20 32	24	02 24	23	08 11	23	13 58
September	Libra	23	17 45	23	23 38	23	05 26	23	11 13
October	Scorpio	24	02 36	24	08 29	23	14 18	23	20 07
November	Sagittarius	22	23 44	23	05 36	22	11 25	22	17 17
December	Capricorn	22	12 50	22	18 37	22	00 27	22	06 22

In the Month of	The Sun entered	1938 Day	Hr min	1939 Day	Hr min	1940 Day	Hr min	1941 Day	Hr min
January	Aquarius	20	16 59	20	22 51	21	04 44	20	10 34
February	Pisces	19	07 20	19	13 09	19	19 04	19	00 56
March	Aries	21	06 43	21	12 28	20	18 24	21	00 20
April	Taurus	20	18 15	20	23 55	20	05 51	20	11 50
May	Gemini	21	17 50	21	23 27	21	05 23	21	11 23
June	Cancer	22	02 03	22	07 39	21	13 36	21	19 33
July	Leo	23	12 57	23	18 37	23	00 34	23	06 26
August	Virgo	23	19 46	24	01 31	23	07 29	23	13 17
September	Libra	23	17 00	23	22 50	23	04 46	23	10 33
October	Scorpio	24	01 54	24	07 46	23	13 39	23	19 27
November	Sagittarius	22	23 06	23	04 59	22	10 49	22	16 38
December	Capricorn	22	12 14	22	18 06	21	23 55	22	05 44

In the Month of	The Sun entered	1942 Day	Hr min	1943 Day	Hr min	1944 Day	Hr min	1945 Day	Hr min
January	Aquarius	20	16 24	20	22 19	21	04 07	20	09 54
February	Pisces	19	06 47	19	12 40	19	18 27	19	00 15
March	Aries	21	06 11	21	12 03	20	17 49	20	23 37
April	Taurus	20	17 39	20	23 31	20	05 18	20	11 07
May	Gemini	21	17 09	21	23 03	21	04 51	21	10 40
June	Cancer	22	01 16	22	07 12	21	13 02	21	18 52
July	Leo	23	12 07	23	18 04	22	23 56	23	05 45
August	Virgo	23	18 58	24	00 55	23	06 47	23	12 35
September	Libra	23	16 17	23	22 12	23	04 02	23	09 50
October	Scorpio	24	01 15	24	07 08	23	12 56	23	18 44
November	Sagittarius	22	22 31	23	04 22	22	10 08	22	15 55
December	Capricorn	22	11 40	22	17 29	21	23 15	22	05 04

In the Month of	The Sun entered	1946 Day	Hr min	1947 Day	Hr min	1948 Day	Hr min	1949 Day	Hr min
January	Aquarius	20	15 45	20	21 32	21	03 19	20	09 09
February	Pisces	19	06 09	19	11 52	19	17 37	18	23 27
March	Aries	21	05 33	21	11 13	20	16 57	20	22 48
April	Taurus	20	17 02	20	22 39	20	04 25	20	10 17
May	Gemini	21	16 34	21	22 09	21	03 58	21	09 51
June	Cancer	22	00 44	22	06 19	21	12 11	21	18 03
July	Leo	23	11 37	23	17 14	22	23 08	23	04 57
August	Virgo	23	18 26	24	00 09	23	06 03	23	11 48
September	Libra	23	15 41	23	21 29	23	03 22	23	09 06
October	Scorpio	24	00 35	24	06 26	23	12 18	23	18 03
November	Sagittarius	22	21 47	23	03 38	22	09 29	22	15 16
December	Capricorn	22	10 54	22	16 43	21	22 33	22	04 23

In the Month of	The Sun entered	1950 Day	Hr min	1951 Day	Hr min	1952 Day	Hr min	1953 Day	Hr min
January	Aquarius	20	15 00	20	20 52	21	02 39	20	08 22
February	Pisces	19	05 18	19	11 10	19	16 57	18	22 41
March	Aries	21	04 35	21	10 26	20	16 14	20	22 00
April	Taurus	20	15 59	20	21 48	20	03 37	20	09 25
May	Gemini	21	15 27	21	21 15	21	03 04	21	08 53
June	Cancer	21	23 36	22	05 25	21	11 12	21	17 00
July	Leo	23	10 30	23	16 21	22	22 07	23	03 52
August	Virgo	23	17 23	23	23 16	23	05 03	23	10 45
September	Libra	23	14 44	23	20 37	23	02 24	23	08 06
October	Scorpio	23	23 45	24	05 36	23	11 22	23	17 06
November	Sagittarius	22	21 03	23	02 51	22	08 36	22	14 22
December	Capricorn	22	10 14	22	16 00	21	21 43	22	03 32

In the Month of	The Sun entered	1954 Day	Hr min	1955 Day	Hr min	1956 Day	Hr min	1957 Day	Hr min
January	Aquarius	20	14 11	20	20 02	21	01 49	20	07 39
February	Pisces	19	04 32	19	10 19	19	16 05	18	21 58
March	Aries	21	03 53	21	09 35	20	15 20	20	21 16
April	Taurus	20	15 19	20	20 58	20	02 43	20	08 41
May	Gemini	21	14 47	21	20 24	21	02 12	21	08 10
June	Cancer	21	22 54	22	04 31	22	10 24	21	16 20
July	Leo	23	09 45	23	15 25	22	21 20	23	03 15
August	Virgo	23	16 36	23	22 19	23	04 15	23	10 08
September	Libra	23	13 55	23	19 41	23	01 35	23	07 26
October	Scorpio	23	22 57	24	04 43	23	10 35	23	16 24
November	Sagittarius	22	20 14	23	02 01	22	07 50	22	13 39
December	Capricorn	22	09 25	22	15 11	21	21 00	22	02 49

In the Month of	The Sun entered	1958 Day	Hr min	1959 Day	Hr min	1960 Day	Hr min	1961 Day	Hr min
January	Aquarius	20	13 29	20	19 19	21	01 10	20	07 01
February	Pisces	19	03 49	19	09 38	19	15 26	18	21 17
March	Aries	21	03 06	21	08 55	20	14 43	20	20 32
April	Taurus	20	14 27	20	20 16	20	02 06	20	07 55
May	Gemini	21	13 51	21	19 42	21	01 33	21	07 22
June	Cancer	21	21 57	22	03 50	21	09 42	21	15 30
July	Leo	23	08 51	23	14 45	22	20 37	23	02 24
August	Virgo	23	15 46	23	21 44	23	03 35	23	09 19
September	Libra	23	13 09	23	19 09	23	00 59	23	06 43
October	Scorpio	23	22 12	24	04 11	23	10 02	23	15 48
November	Sagittarius	22	19 29	23	01 27	22	07 19	22	13 08
December	Capricorn	22	08 40	22	14 35	21	20 26	22	02 20

In the Month of	The Sun entered	1962 Day	Hr min	1963 Day	Hr min	1964 Day	Hr min	1965 Day	Hr min
January	Aquarius	20	12 58	20	18 54	21	00 41	20	06 29
February	Pisces	19	03 15	19	09 09	19	14 58	18	20 48
March	Aries	21	02 30	21	08 20	20	14 10	20	20 05
April	Taurus	20	13 51	20	19 36	20	01 27	20	07 26
May	Gemini	21	13 16	21	18 58	21	00 50	21	06 50
June	Cancer	21	21 24	22	03 04	21	08 57	21	14 56
July	Leo	23	08 18	23	13 59	22	19 53	23	01 48
August	Virgo	23	15 13	23	20 58	23	02 51	23	08 43
September	Libra	23	12 35	23	18 24	23	00 17	23	06 06
October	Scorpio	23	21 40	24	03 29	23	09 21	23	15 10
November	Sagittarius	22	19 02	23	00 50	22	06 39	22	12 29
December	Capricorn	22	08 16	22	14 02	21	19 50	22	01 41

In the Month of	The Sun entered	1966 Day	Hr min	1967 Day	Hr min	1968 Day	Hr min	1969 Day	Hr min
January	Aquarius	20	12 20	20	18 08	20	23 54	20	05 39
February	Pisces	19	02 38	19	08 24	19	14 09	18	19 55
March	Aries	21	01 53	21	07 37	20	13 22	20	19 08
April	Taurus	20	13 11	20	18 55	20	00 41	20	06 27
May	Gemini	21	12 32	21	18 18	21	00 06	21	05 50
June	Cancer	21	20 33	22	02 23	21	08 13	21	13 55
July	Leo	23	07 23	23	13 16	22	19 07	23	00 48
August	Virgo	23	14 18	23	20 13	23	02 03	23	07 44
September	Libra	23	11 43	23	17 38	22	23 26	23	05 07
October	Scorpio	23	20 51	24	02 44	23	08 30	23	14 11
November	Sagittarius	22	18 14	23	00 05	22	05 49	22	11 31
December	Capricorn	22	07 29	22	13 17	21	19 00	22	00 44

In the Month of	The Sun entered	1970 Day	Hr min	1971 Day	Hr min	1972 Day	Hr min	1973 Day	Hr min
January	Aquarius	20	11 24	20	17 13	20	22 59	20	04 49
February	Pisces	19	01 42	19	07 27	19	13 12	18	19 01
March	Aries	21	00 57	21	06 38	20	12 22	20	18 13
April	Taurus	20	12 15	20	17 54	19	23 37	20	05 30
May	Gemini	21	11 37	21	17 15	20	22 59	21	04 54
June	Cancer	21	19 43	22	01 20	21	07 06	21	13 01
July	Leo	23	06 37	23	12 15	22	18 03	22	23 56
August	Virgo	23	13 34	23	19 15	23	01 03	23	06 54
September	Libra	23	10 59	23	16 45	22	22 33	23	04 21
October	Scorpio	23	20 04	24	01 53	23	07 42	23	13 30
November	Sagittarius	22	17 25	22	23 14	22	05 03	22	10 54
December	Capricorn	22	06 36	22	12 24	21	18 13	22	00 08

In the Month of	The Sun entered	1974 Day	Hr min	1975 Day	Hr min	1976 Day	Hr min	1977 Day	Hr min
January	Aquarius	20	10 46	20	16 37	20	22 25	20	04 15
February	Pisces	19	00 59	19	06 50	19	12 40	18	18 31
March	Aries	21	00 07	21	05 57	20	11 50	20	17 42
April	Taurus	20	11 19	20	17 07	19	23 03	20	04 57
May	Gemini	21	10 36	21	16 24	20	22 21	21	04 14
June	Cancer	21	18 38	22	00 26	21	06 24	21	12 14
July	Leo	23	05 30	23	11 22	22	17 19	22	23 04
August	Virgo	23	12 29	23	18 24	23	00 18	23	06 01
September	Libra	23	09 59	23	15 55	22	21 48	23	03 30
October	Scorpio	23	19 11	24	01 06	23	06 58	23	12 41
November	Sagittarius	22	16 39	22	22 31	22	04 22	22	10 07
December	Capricorn	22	05 56	22	11 46	21	17 36	21	23 24

In the Month of	The Sun entered	1978 Day	Hr min	1979 Day	Hr min	1980 Day	Hr min	1981 Day	Hr min
January	Aquarius	20	10 04	20	16 00	20	21 49	20	03 36
February	Pisces	19	00 21	19	06 13	19	12 02	18	17 52
March	Aries	20	23 34	21	05 22	20	11 10	20	17 03
April	Taurus	20	10 50	20	16 35	19	22 23	20	04 19
May	Gemini	21	10 08	21	15 54	20	21 42	21	03 39
June	Cancer	21	18 10	21	23 56	21	05 47	21	11 40
July	Leo	23	05 00	23	10 49	22	16 42	22	22 40
August	Virgo	23	11 57	23	17 47	22	23 41	23	05 38
September	Libra	23	09 26	23	15 17	22	21 09	23	03 05
October	Scorpio	23	18 37	24	00 28	23	06 18	23	12 13
November	Sagittarius	22	16 05	22	21 54	22	03 42	22	09 36
December	Capricorn	22	05 21	22	11 10	21	16 56	21	22 51

In the Month of	The Sun entered	1982 Day	Hr min	1983 Day	Hr min	1984 Day	Hr min	1985 Day	Hr min
January	Aquarius	20	09 31	20	15 17	20	21 05	20	02 58
February	Pisces	18	23 47	19	05 31	19	11 16	18	17 08
March	Aries	20	22 56	21	04 39	20	10 25	20	16 14
April	Taurus	20	10 08	20	15 50	19	21 38	20	03 26
May	Gemini	21	09 23	21	15 06	20	20 58	21	02 43
June	Cancer	21	17 23	21	23 09	21	05 02	21	10 44
July	Leo	23	04 16	23	10 04	22	15 58	22	21 37
August	Virgo	23	11 15	23	17 08	22	23 00	23	04 36
September	Libra	23	08 47	23	14 42	22	20 33	23	02 08
October	Scorpio	23	17 58	23	23 55	23	05 46	23	11 22
November	Sagittarius	22	15 24	22	21 19	22	03 11	22	08 51
December	Capricorn	22	04 39	22	10 30	21	16 23	21	22 08

In the Month of	The Sun entered	1986 Day	Hr min	1987 Day	Hr min	1988 Day	Hr min	1989 Day	Hr min
January	Aquarius	20	08 47	20	14 41	20	20 25	20	02 07
February	Pisces	18	22 58	19	04 50	19	10 36	18	16 21
March	Aries	20	22 03	21	03 52	20	09 39	20	15 29
April	Taurus	20	09 12	20	14 58	19	20 45	20	02 39
May	Gemini	21	08 28	21	14 10	20	19 57	21	01 54
June	Cancer	21	16 30	21	22 11	21	03 57	21	09 53
July	Leo	23	03 25	23	09 06	22	14 51	22	20 46
August	Virgo	23	10 26	23	16 10	22	21 54	23	03 46
September	Libra	23	07 59	23	13 46	22	19 29	23	01 20
October	Scorpio	23	17 15	23	23 01	23	04 44	23	10 36
November	Sagittarius	22	14 45	22	20 30	22	02 12	22	08 05
December	Capricorn	22	04 03	22	09 46	21	15 28	21	21 22

In the Month of	The Sun entered	1990 Day	Hr min	1991 Day	Hr min	1992 Day	Hr min	1993 Day	Hr min
January	Aquarius	20	08 02	20	13 48	20	19 33	20	01 23
February	Pisces	18	22 14	19	03 59	19	09 44	18	15 36
March	Aries	20	21 19	21	03 02	20	08 48	20	14 41
April	Taurus	20	08 27	20	14 09	19	19 57	20	01 49
May	Gemini	21	07 37	21	13 20	20	19 12	21	01 02
June	Cancer	21	15 33	22	21 19	21	03 14	21	09 00
July	Leo	23	02 22	23	08 11	22	14 09	22	19 51
August	Virgo	23	09 21	23	15 13	22	21 10	23	02 51
September	Libra	23	06 56	23	12 48	22	18 43	23	00 23
October	Scorpio	23	16 14	23	22 05	23	03 57	23	09 38
November	Sagittarius	22	13 47	22	19 36	22	01 26	22	07 07
December	Capricorn	22	03 07	22	08 54	21	14 44	21	20 26